WHAT WE <u>DO</u> KNOW ABOUT HEART ATTACKS

WHAT WE DO KNOW
ABOUT HEART ATTACKS

JOHN W. GOFMAN, M.D.

Professor of Medical Physics
University of California
Berkeley

G. P. PUTNAM'S SONS, NEW YORK

© 1958 by John W. Gofman

Published simultaneously in the Dominion of
Canada by Longmans, Green & Company, Toronto.

Library of Congress Catalog Card Number: 58-11669

MANUFACTURED IN THE UNITED STATES OF AMERICA

Contents

Introduction

It is rare to encounter a family in our society that has not had personal experience with heart attacks, either directly or among close friends. The frequency of occurrence of heart attacks in our population is so high that this disease now outranks all others by a very wide margin as the major cause of serious disability and death. This is amply illustrated by our vital statistics, which reveal that heart attacks account for approximately three times as many deaths as *all forms of cancer combined.*

At one time heart attacks were considered a more or less inevitable consequence of growing old. Erroneously, some still think this is the case. Indeed, there is prevalent some opinion that since we must die in some way, heart attacks—usually sudden—may represent a relatively favorable way to leave this world. The basic premises underlying such thinking are wholly incorrect. Heart attacks *do* occur with increasing frequency with increasing age, but they also occur all too frequently early in life, especially in men, when individuals are at the height of their productivity and usefulness to society. Forty- and fifty-year-old men, in whom a vast number of heart attacks occur each year, can hardly by any stretch of the imagination be considered "old" men. Hence we can safely say that even though age may be one factor in the disease, it is not by any means the only one. Certainly some more satisfactory explanation than aging alone is required to understand the high incidence of heart attacks in men under fifty and even under forty years of age.

A prime feature of the entire phenomenon of heart attacks, and probably its most terrifying aspect, is its *suddenness of occurrence*. A person, by ordinary techniques of medical examination, may have been pronounced in excellent health one day, one hour, or even one minute before a fatal heart attack. This aspect of the disease has been brought into sharp relief by the following statement of the cardiologist for a large life insurance company: "It is most disturbing that men can have a fatal heart attack before the ink has dried on a large life insurance policy that has just been issued them."

It is quite understandable, then, that repeatedly the question is raised by industrial chiefs, military leaders, and the heads of governments: "Is there no way to predict who the likely candidates are for the development of disabling or fatal coronary heart disease *before* the sudden occurrence of a heart attack?" Obviously a basic prerequisite for a positive approach to the all-important problem of *prevention* of heart attacks is some method for preselection of those individuals who carry an unduly large risk of subsequent development of heart attacks.

Or, if heart attacks cannot be completely prevented, there does exist the prospect, by early recognition of those especially prone, of postponing the disease to a much later period in life. This question of whether prediction of the hazard of coronary heart attacks is possible in an individual deserves most serious consideration and thoughtful reply inasmuch as it represents one of the most important questions facing our adult population today. Yet in widespread lay and medical sources bland, platitudinous replies have been repeatedly issued in apparent total oblivion of a rather enormous pool of sound scientific information, won at great cost, upon which a thoughtful reply might be based.

Comments from uninformed sources are steadily made to the effect that the basis for heart attacks remains a complete mystery and that prediction of the disease in advance of its overt presence is impossible. Such comments are made in spite of the fact that all of the scientific evidence, accumulated through the efforts of numerous investigators, contradicts these statements completely. It would thus appear that the average intelligent layman might want explained in familiar terms what we *do* know today about heart attacks, their real nature, and their predictability, since in actual fact a great deal of the "mystery" surrounding heart attacks has been cleared away in recent years.

It is the author's purpose to provide here the evidence that has been solidly accumulated concerning heart attacks, their basis, the prospects for prediction of those carrying a high risk of the disease, and the directions in which such evidence suggests that resolution of the problem of heart attack prevention may lie. This information, translated into usual terms, will, it is hoped, prove helpful to the intelligent layman who is interested in this problem but who does not himself have known heart disease. It should also be helpful to the person with heart disease who wishes to have a clearer picture of what this disease truly is and the why and wherefore of some of the treatment and preventive measures advised by physicians.

CHAPTER 1

The Heart Attack and Its Underlying Basis

Although there is some loose usage of the term *heart attack*, there is almost universal concurrence by laymen and physicians alike that this term denotes a specific medical entity. This medical entity may present itself in a particular patient overtly in one of several forms with respect to the actual signs and symptoms noted. Depending upon these signs and symptoms, several different terms have been utilized to describe the disease, such as *coronary occlusion*, *coronary thrombosis*, *angina pectoris*, *myocardial infarction*, *coronary disease*, or simply *heart attack*. It is immediately to be noted that the word *coronary* occurs with great frequency in the description of the disease entity, and aptly so, for coronary is the name applied to those arteries (blood vessels) which supply the heart muscle itself with a blood supply. Such a blood supply is, for the heart as for other organs, vital in the provision of nutrition, oxygen, and as a means for the disposal of the waste products of metabolism. In recognition of this vital role of supplying blood to the heart muscle, the vessels performing this task are regarded as the "crown" arteries, or "coronary" arteries.

Essentially, the heart is an organized mass of specialized muscle tissue which performs a pumping function. Even though large volumes of blood are of course present within the chambers of the heart, little if any significant nutrition comes directly to the critical heart muscle through the walls of the heart's chambers. Such nutrition comes via the branches of the coronary arteries, which are imbedded in the heart's surface and which send a multitude of small branches into the various regions of the heart muscle itself. Further, the heart muscle possesses very little reserve of nutrients and oxygen, and hence depends for its integrity and life upon an uninterrupted supply of nutrition and oxygen through the blood supply provided by the coronary arteries. Should this supply of blood by way of the coronary arteries be significantly diminished or cut off entirely, the heart muscle is placed in imminent danger of its survival as a living, functioning tissue. As will be elaborated later, it is known that the blood supply to some part of the heart muscle can and does become compromised by closure of a small or large branch of the coronary arterial tree. Such an event is essentially what provides the immediate setting for a heart attack, since the heart muscle cannot survive long without restoration of its blood supply. Fortunately, in many instances, the branch of the coronary arteries which closes down is a relatively small one, so that the area of heart muscle which suffers is in turn small. Such an area of heart muscle may be injured sufficiently to die, or it may survive in an injured form.

If the area of heart muscle so injured or killed is small, nature's reparative processes may enable the patient to survive through the mechanism of gradual replacement of the dead or dying heart muscle by a tough, fibrous scar. Even though this fibrous tissue scar cannot aid in the pumping function of the heart, it does prevent catastrophe in the form of an actual rupture, or "blowout," of the heart wall itself. It is remarkable and indeed fortunate that an individual can live, with minimum limitation of activity, even with *several* such scars of previous heart attacks. The reason why the early days and weeks following a heart attack are so critical is that during this period "blowout" is a great danger, since several weeks are required for the formation of a firm scar (the fibrous tissue replacement for the injured or dead heart muscle). Thus complete bed rest with an absolute minimum of exertion is generally advised for the early period following a heart attack.

All the foregoing considerations refer to the situation which exists when the branch of the coronary arteries closing down is a relatively small one. If, in contrast, a somewhat larger branch of the coronary arteries closes down, the consequences can be much more disastrous. In such an event the area of heart muscle deprived of its blood supply is much larger. If this area is large enough and the damage to it severe enough, there may be interference with the rhythmic impulse of the heartbeat itself, so that a highly irregular heart action may establish itself. Certain of these highly irregular heart rhythms may be incompatible with the pumping function of the heart, and sudden death may occur. Or, if death does not occur, the area of heart muscle involved may be large enough that the danger of rupture or "blowout" of the heart wall is enormously increased, an event which also leads to death. Even if an adequate fibrous tissue scar replacement forms, it may be so large that the remaining heart muscle cannot adequately carry the load as a pump, with the result that the patient may become an invalid or die of a disorder known as *heart failure*. In essence, heart failure means that the heart can no longer function adequately as a pump.

Any of these events occurring in the heart muscle is a consequence of a compromised, inadequate blood supply to the heart muscle itself. It goes without saying that once an accident has occurred, leading to a markedly diminished blood supply to the heart, all attention must rightly be focused upon efforts to protect the life of the victim through the critical days and weeks that follow. For this patient nothing is momentarily of greater importance. However, any intelligent person who has suffered such a catastrophe, or who knows someone who has, may be expected to ask a very important and very pertinent question: "Why did the coronary artery branch close down and thus deprive the heart muscle of its blood supply?" A brief consideration will reveal that this question is the very crux of the entire problem of heart attacks, for if the artery had never closed down, there would have been no injury to heart muscle and hence no heart attack. If we are to achieve *prevention* of heart attacks, we must understand, above all, the way in which arteries close down and the reason or reasons why they close down. If we concern ourselves primarily with the problem of what to do *after* a person has suffered a heart attack, we are in a very real sense "locking the barn *long* after the horse has been stolen."

What is the real nature of the closing down (or *occlusion*, in medical parlance) of the coronary arteries which supply the heart muscle with blood? Broadly speaking, there are two major types of closure, one that occurs slowly and progressively over a period of many months or years and a second which occurs rapidly over a short period, probably of minutes or hours. Furthermore, it is of the greatest interest and importance that the rapid form of closure occurs almost wholly in those parts of the coronary arteries which are already suffering from the effects of the slow form of closure or narrowing. The rapid type of closure is in general the result of clotting, or solidification, of the blood within the arterial channel, this artery having in general already been partially narrowed or closed by the slow type of closure. Since this is the case, the major problem underlying the occurrence of heart attacks is *the slow type of narrowing or closure of the coronary arteries*. There can be little doubt that it is to this disease process that most of our attention must necessarily be directed if our goal is an ultimate reduction in the mortality rate from heart attacks.

The slow type of narrowing or closure of the coronary arteries —which occurs probably over months, years, and even decades —has been described by various names both in the medical and nonmedical literature. Among the prominent descriptions of the process which results in narrowing or slow closure of the coronary vessels are such terms as *arteriosclerosis* and *atherosclerosis*. These somewhat formidable terms actually have rather simple meanings and origins. *Sclerosis* is a general medical term meaning "hardening." When arteries become narrower they do so in part by a firm overgrowth in their walls of fibrous tissue and in part by a deposition of lime salts (calcium salts). Thus the term *sclerosis* has come to be an apt description of a major part of the process. The *arterio-* part of the name of the process simply refers to the fact that the sclerosis, or hardening, is going on in a blood vessel of the arterial type, rather than, for example, in a vein. The designation *atheromeans* "porridge" or "gruel." This term was applied to the arterial disease because, as the artery narrows, part of the wall becomes loaded with a fatty, yellowish material which, to the earlier pathologists, bore a resemblance to gruel or mush.

Actually, arteriosclerosis and atherosclerosis cannot be sharply differentiated as separate entities and indeed the aspects of the disease inferred by both names are generally present in the same region of any artery considered. What we must understand by both terms is that a process (or several processes) goes on in the arterial wall leading to its slow narrowing, and that this includes some hardening due to fibrous tissue overgrowth, lime salt deposition, and involves a fatty deposition resembling gruel. All of this combined is the real essence of what is popularly known as "hardening of the arteries." Although much discussion and controversy have centered around the question of whether the hardening or the fatty deposition is most important, this has in large measure represented an academic exercise of little merit. The vast bulk of the evidence suggests that the most crucial feature is actually the gradual narrowing of the arteries that occurs plus the fact that such narrowed arteries are inordinately susceptible to the clotting of blood within them. This latter event is so often the rapid occurrence that immediately precedes the heart attack. Since clotting of blood in blood vessel is known medically as *thrombosis*, we can readily understand why heart attacks are often referred to as coronary thrombosis.

The important sequence of events may now be summarized. For some reason (to be discussed in detail later) arteries undergo a gradual narrowing by the processes known as arteriosclerosis and atherosclerosis. This gradual narrowing plus, in many instances, a rapid narrowing due to blood clotting (and solidification) within the narrowed artery finally results in a marked decrease in the blood supply to the heart muscle. Such a decrease in blood supply to the heart may seriously damage the part of the heart muscle involved, with that disastrous consequence known as the heart attack. The life or death of the patient then hinges upon the extent of the damage and the extent to which nature's reparative processes can help. It should be clear, therefore, that an attack upon the problem of this form of heart disease (the major form) must essentially be an attack upon the problem of the gradual narrowing of the coronary arteries due to arteriosclerosis and atherosclerosis. If the gradual narrowing of the arteries could be prevented, the subsequent events would not occur, and heart attacks (and their enormous toll in health and life) would become rare to the point of vanishing.

CHAPTER **2**

The Search for a Causative Factor in Coronary Artery Narrowing

In Chapter 1 it was pointed out that the major factor underlying heart attacks is a gradual narrowing of the heart's own
arteries, the coronary arteries, by disease processes known as
arteriosclerosis and atherosclerosis. The term *disease processes*
is used advisedly, since for many years there existed a school
of thought in medicine which held that arteriosclerosis and
atherosclerosis were perfectly normal processes that could be
regarded as simply "part and parcel of growing old."

If this were simply an academic consideration, one would
hardly care whether some people chose to regard these processes as just part of growing old. But it must be stated that
the existence of this view has served as one of the greatest
deterrents to progress in the field of heart disease that has yet
appeared. For, if arteriosclerosis and atherosclerosis are truly
part and parcel of growing old, there is little we should do
about them but to accept them gracefully and with resignation.
No serious student of the problem of coronary heart disease
can any longer countenance this outdated view. A multitude
of types of evidence has been accumulated which demon-
strates clearly the erroneous nature of this concept. The all-too-
frequent occurrence of severe coronary artery narrowing (and

7

fatal heart attacks) in otherwise robust men in their twenties and thirties argues strongly against the "growing old" concept. Furthermore, it is now well known that many people reach their seventies and eighties and at death (from other causes) show very little involvement of their coronary arteries with arteriosclerosis or atherosclerosis. All the evidence suggests that arteriosclerosis and atherosclerosis and coronary artery narrowing represent facets of disease processes that are by no means confined only to the aging or aged and that should under no circumstances be regarded as inevitable.

Our quest, then, is for an answer to the question "What is the basis for the disease which results in narrowing of the coronary arteries?" With respect to any disease, the search for an underlying basis or cause generally poses a monumental problem. Especially is this the case for a disease process that goes on insidiously for many years without being obviously felt until it announces its presence in severe degree by the occurrence of a heart attack. We know that hard and long efforts were necessary to learn the bases for the relative handful of diseases for which the causes are known. The realization is sobering that there are many more diseases for which the causes are unknown.

Certain approaches do, however, suggest themselves in the endeavor to seek out a cause or basis for coronary artery narrowing. Following classical lines of investigation, one may search for an infectious agent such as a bacterium or a virus, or for a dietary deficiency such as a vitamin deficiency, or for some toxic or noxious agent in the environment. To date the efforts to find some such single cause of arteriosclerosis or atherosclerosis of the coronary arteries have been unrewarding, although this does not by any means rule out a positive finding in one of these directions in the future. Failing directly in the effort to find a single cause along classical lines, one may marshal the existing evidence with respect to the disease in the hope that certain clues can be put together to point in a definitive direction to the basis or cause of the disease under study. This latter approach has been very fruitful in pinpointing the underlying basis for atherosclerosis and arteriosclerosis of the coronary arteries. In this type of approach no evidence can be overlooked, even though the sources of information may be quite diverse and seemingly unrelated. Indeed, overlooking some particular type of evidence bearing upon the disease may lose for the inquirer precisely the lead which would have led to great clarification. Since we can afford to overlook no evidence, let us consider the various types of information at our disposal concerning heart attacks, which must ultimately be integrated into a composite whole.

First, *who* develops coronary artery hardening and narrowing and their consequence, heart attacks? It is amazing what a clue the answer to this question has represented. We can say broadly that, *on the average*, there is more coronary artery disease narrowing and there are more frequent heart attacks with *increasing chronological age*. Heart attacks due to coronary artery narrowing are very rare in childhood, although they may occur in selected instances which will be considered later. Heart attacks do become progressively more frequent with the passage of each decade of life beyond childhood. By this we mean that out of 1000 persons there will be a greater number of heart attacks per year for thirty-five-year-olds than for twenty-five-year-olds, for forty-five-year-olds than for thirty-five-year-olds, and so on for each succeeding decade of life. Thus the evidence is good that age is unquestionably a factor in both coronary artery narrowing and in the occurrence of heart attacks. But it is important to avoid the pitfall of making the wholly unreasonable and unjustifiable assumption that age is the only factor or even by any means the most important factor involved. That age is not the *only* factor is nicely contradicted by several facets of evidence: (1) Severe coronary artery narrowing can and does occur in some youthful individuals in the 'teens, twenties, and thirties. (2) Many persons in the later decades of life (for example, the seventies) are relatively free of this disease process. (3) Even if we compare individuals at a given age (for example, forty years of age) and limit our observations to one sex, one occupational category, one race, one height, one weight, and comparable with regard to many other features, we still will find that certain of these individuals show extensive coronary artery narrowing, others moderate narrowing, and some will show almost none of this disease process. This finding, it is to be noted, can be made where *all* the individuals are of exactly the *same chronological* age. How then shall we interpret the clue of age? There can be no denial of the average increase of coronary artery narrowing with increase of age, but there are so many exceptions of marked degree to this average trend that we must conclude that age is one factor but only one of the factors that operate. The age effect can be and is in many individuals overshadowed by some other factor or factors. We shall return later to this question of the age factor, for considered in the light of many other findings it enables us to clarify many otherwise apparently paradoxical findings.

Going on with the question of who develops coronary artery narrowing and coronary heart attacks, we come upon the remarkable observation that in practically every country where the problem has been given serious attention it has been found that men of a particular age, especially in the age groups below sixty years, are more likely to develop heart attacks than are women of the same age. In the thirties, it appears that men are at least four or five times as likely to develop heart attacks as are women. As confirmation it has also been found in the study of the coronary arteries of persons who have died in accidents that there is more of the coronary artery narrowing to be noted in the average man of thirty-five years of age than in the average woman of the same age. Again this clue is not an all-or-none clue. Some women do develop extensive coronary artery narrowing early in life and do have heart attacks, and many men of the same age have much less coronary artery narrowing than *some* women. But the average trend, both with respect to extent of coronary artery narrowing and heart attack rate, is unmistakably higher in men than in women. Again, a relatively simple observation provides us with information of enormous value in our search, and it becomes apparent that somewhere in our over-all picture of the disease this clue—the difference between men and women—must be put into its proper place.

What else do we know of *who* develops this disease? It has been observed long ago that certain families seem inordinately prone to the development of early and severe narrowing of their coronary arteries and to the occurrence of serious or fatal heart attacks early in life. In some of these families one may discover upon questioning that, of three brothers and two sisters in a family, all suffered one or more heart attacks before the age of forty years, with some having had their heart attacks in the twenties. For so many young individuals in a family to suffer heart attacks before forty years of age, by the laws of chance alone, is so improbable that there can be no question that these families must have something operating to produce such a dismal picture with respect to the outlook for heart disease. So well accepted is the knowledge that certain families seem inordinately susceptible to heart attacks that some wags have facetiously remarked that the best way to avoid coronary disease is to choose one's ancestors carefully. But, as with the other clues, this one is not universal either, for there exist many families with a history of longevity in which one member of the family may suffer from early extensive coronary artery narrowing and an early heart attack while other members of the family do not. The observation of the positive familial relationship in some cases is, however, a solidly based one and is therefore one of the definitive pieces of the puzzle requiring ultimate assembly. Much is now understood concerning the mechanism by which such familial factors operate; this will be elaborated later in this book.

Other types of evidence have been brought to bear upon the question of *who* has coronary artery narrowing and heart attacks. One prominent type of evidence has arisen out of geographical studies of the incidence of the disease. In certain countries coronary artery narrowing and the occurrence of heart attacks is extensive, as it is in the United States, where the problem is so serious as to constitute our number one medical problem in adults. Elsewhere in the world there are countries where narrowing of the coronary arteries proceeds much more slowly and where the occurrence of heart attacks is so relatively infrequent that medical authorities hardly consider heart disease of this type worthy of more than passing comment. The geographical clue is of undoubted importance, although it is evident that there are many factors which differ from one country to another, such as race, climatic factors, dietary factors, prevalence of pestilence, and a host of others. Yet it turns out that it is possible to find certain central features that distinguish persons in one country from those in another, such features probably being of direct importance in predicting why the incidence of coronary heart disease differs in almost any two countries under consideration.

Other features may now be considered in our search for clues. One that interests people a great deal is the possible relationship of overweight to the development of coronary artery narrowing and to the hazard of occurrence of heart attacks. It can be stated first that all observers know that heart attacks are limited neither to the fat nor to the thin. Thus, as with so many other factors, overweight cannot possibly be an absolute criterion. However, very impressive evidence indeed is available that incriminates overweight in the development of coronary artery narrowing and as a factor in increasing the risk of heart attacks. Foremost among such evidence is that developed by the life insurance companies in observing the occurrence rate of coronary heart attacks of policyholders over many years. They have found, in virtually indisputable studies, that the rate of occurrence of heart attacks was strikingly greater, on the average, in their overweight policyholders than in those who were not overweight. Pathologists studying the arteries of persons who had died of a variety of causes have also shown that there is more coronary artery narrowing, on the average, in the overweight than in those not overweight. Popularly, and in many medical circles, it is felt that the explanation for excessive heart disease in the overweight is a simple one. We are often treated to the analogy of a fat man being the same as a thin one except that the fat man is carrying a large suitcase filled with 50 pounds of fat. This, it is stated, presents a large burden to the heart. Scientifically, however, it is amazing how little evidence exists to support this "excess baggage" concept of the relationship of overweight to heart disease. On the other hand, the *existence* of a relationship of overweight to excessive heart disease is clear. This clue, together with others, does allow for a great insight into the probable mechanisms that account for the observed relationship, together with some very hopeful prospects for utilizing the information in the prevention of heart attacks.

High blood pressure is very commonly associated in the minds of both layman and physician with coronary heart attacks. Some people have erroneously considered arteriosclerosis and high blood pressure as one and the same disease. It has become quite clear from relatively recent studies that definite relationship does exist, in an average sense, between blood pressure levels and coronary heart attacks. Attention to this relationship may help in understanding some otherwise obscure features of the disease and in providing some useful approaches to prevention and treatment of the disease.

Numerous other features have been under study in the effort to seek out clues to the basis for coronary heart attacks. Among these are such questions as composition of the diet, cigarette smoking habits, occupational groups, body types, extent of exercise, hormonal balance, and the "stress and strain of modern living." Some of these have been quite rewarding and have made a great contribution to our understanding of the nature of the disease; others still elude us, at least in part, often because of great difficulty in making any quantitative estimations that can be used in analysis of the evidence.

In summary, it can be stated that even though no simple disease-causing agent such as a bacterium, a virus, or a toxic material has been found for coronary artery narrowing (and for heart attacks, which represent a consequence of such narrowing), we are certainly not without a host of valuable clues, each based upon solidly founded and documented scientific information. When such a situation arises involving a set of individual clues, there are two possibilities: either all the clues are wholly unrelated to each other, or several (possibly all) may be presenting to us different facets of a single important basic aspect of the disease. If it turned out that all the clues were unrelated, the study of the disease would be extremely difficult, although one would still have to go forward to evaluate each clue and assess its role in the disease.

In the case of coronary artery hardening and coronary heart attacks, it has now become evident that most of the clues described above are indeed closely related and intertwined. When placed in their proper perspective and interpreted, it is found not only that we obtain a very reasonable integrated picture concerning heart attacks, but also that the various facets prove complementary to each other. This greatly increases our confidence that the understanding derived must be a fruitful one, worth applying in the effort to make a serious attack upon the problem of minimizing or preventing coronary heart disease. Attainment of this integrated picture of heart attacks requires that our attention must now be directed to the evidence which leads to an understanding of how all the seemingly unrelated clues described above actually fit together. For this it is essential to consider first the findings that have come from the study of the circulating blood itself, since such studies are central to the understanding of all the facets of coronary artery hardening and coronary heart attacks.

CHAPTER 3

The Importance of the Fatty Substances of the Blood (Lipoproteins) for Heart Attacks

Several seemingly diverse and unrelated clues have been uncovered which bear directly upon the problem of coronary artery narrowing and heart attacks. How do we approach the problem of attempting to mesh these clues together to achieve an understanding of this disease? When we find several features of importance in a disease, at first view unrelated, one reasonable way to proceed is to find out if there exist any denominators common to all or to several of these features. Especially is it desirable that such possible common denominators be measurable and expressible in quantitative terms.

In a new disease problem, it is a matter of no little difficulty to make a decision as to where one should look for possible measurable common denominators. In our present case, one might try by a systematic screening process to measure a great variety of things about people to see if any of them may represent the sought-for common denominator. For example, one might make a measurement, such as the height of a person. Quick consideration of the clues described earlier, however, would show that height can hardly be the factor which will weave any thread of unity through all the evidence at our disposal. Or one might investigate such a factor as the number

16

of red blood cells in the circulating blood. Here again, consideration of the evidence would reveal that this cannot be what is sought. Although in retrospect research workers often like to forget the many blind alleys they have explored, and in their discussions with students make the path that led to a discovery seem like a highly logical sequence of steps, reality is rarely like this. There is always some element of trial and error, some element of hunch, coupled, in the hands of the successful investigator, with "some most reasonable idea of where to look." Our present state of advancement in the integration of the knowledge of heart disease is the result of the trials and errors of many researchers, their hunches, and their reasonable guesses. But it must also be stated that some of the faulty interpretation of research findings made as long ago as twenty-five years served to delay progress in this problem by more than a decade.

Fifty years ago, and in less refined form even a hundred years ago, some reasonable guesses were beginning to be made as to where one should look for common denominators in the problem of coronary artery disease. In the earlier description of the narrowing of the coronary arteries—which sets the stage for ultimate heart attacks—it was noted that some of the material which accumulates on the arterial wall (or in it) and contributes in part to the narrowing is a fatty material, described as resembling gruel or porridge. Investigators asked themselves the reasonable question "What might be the *origin* of the fatty substances which accumulate in the arterial wall and thus contribute in part to the closure of the coronary artery?" One possible answer to this question is that the fatty substances found in the arterial wall are made right there by transformations from other substances (since such transformations can be chemically achieved by living tissues). Indeed, there are today some investigators who are still exploring this idea, although it can be said their work has opened essentially no new vistas for the understanding of coronary disease as yet.

Others suggested early that since the arterial walls are bathed constantly by the blood coursing through the arteries, it might be quite logical to entertain the idea that these fatty substances might get into the arterial walls directly from the blood. How and why fatty substances might go from the blood stream into the arterial wall may be quite a different question to answer. However, the simplicity of the concept of considering the blood as a source of the fatty substances was such that many who prefer to make things as complicated as possible abhorred the idea, and some diehards still do. Nevertheless, the very reasonableness of the concept attracted many students of the disease, who undertook to study the problem from this direction. First it is to be noted that the blood does indeed have several fatty substances dissolved in its fluid portion (the plasma) as well as some fatty substances in the red blood cells. Chemical analyses showed that the major chemical constituents of the fatty materials which accumulate in the arterial wall are *identical with* those of the fatty materials which circulate in the blood. The question then presents itself: "If the fatty substances in the blood do indeed represent the source material for the fatty deposits in the diseased artery wall, why should such deposition occur?"

At this point it is well to recall the observations described earlier which indicate that for the same sex and the same age, two individuals may show vastly different degrees of coronary artery narrowing, and of fatty depositions which are so frequently a part of such narrowing. One possible explanation which was suggested was that some individuals might have greater amounts of fatty substances in the blood than others. Another suggestion was that the fatty substances might be in a different physical or chemical form in the blood of certain people than in that of others. As we shall see later, both suggestions are now regarded as correct, but it is important at this point to trace the development of these lines of reasoning.

Returning to the first suggestion, that individuals with excessive artery hardening might have greater amounts of fatty substances in their blood, the problem that arises is the development of a method for testing the possible validity of this idea. It might appear at first thought that this is an extremely simple idea to test, since all that is necessary is to measure the amount of the fatty substances in an individual's blood and to compare this with the degree of coronary artery narrowing present. But how does one measure the amount of narrowing and hardening of the coronary arteries in the living person who is in a state of apparent health? No method is known that will measure the degree of coronary artery narrowing in a *living* individual, since there is simply no way to look inside the vessels of the heart. This is, in essence, why coronary heart attacks strike without warning. Until the vessel (the coronary artery) closes down enough, especially via the rapid form of closure due to clotting, there is no way, by *usual* tests, to know that a serious degree of this narrowing process has even been going on. To many individuals this would represent a discouraging state of affairs and the problem would be given up as impossible of solution. But this is a highly superficial approach to a challenging problem, and fortunately many investigators did not give up so easily. Here is the concept needing evaluation—that excessive amounts of certain fatty substances of the blood may be related to the development of excessive deposits of fatty substances in the walls of the coronary arteries—but no method exists for measuring the fatty deposits in the arterial walls in the *living* person. Some substitute approach is therefore needed.

Early in the history of the study of coronary artery disease, investigators came up with a logical, brilliant, and extremely simple solution for by-passing the above-described difficulty. They reasoned that since coronary artery narrowing sets the stage for heart attacks, it could be anticipated that a group of persons who had experienced one or more heart attacks would be expected to show more coronary artery narrowing and fatty deposition in the wall of the coronary arteries, on the average, than a group of comparable age and sex where no signs or symptoms of heart disease had become evident. That this reasoning is completely correct has been borne out by several studies of hearts and arteries after death, now classic in the medical literature. These studies show that the degree of coronary artery narrowing and fatty deposition in persons having had a heart attack is strikingly *greater* in degree than in those who died, for example, an accidental death. Thus it was eminently logical to go ahead with studies of the amount of fatty substances in the blood of two groups of persons—those who had survived a heart attack and a group, matched otherwise by age and sex, who had never experienced heart disease to their knowledge. The matching of the groups by age and by sex is very important, since otherwise one is testing several features at once and is led to uninterpretable results. Unfortunately, many medical scientists still do not appreciate this crucial point.

Even by the crude techniques available over twenty-five years ago for measuring the amounts of the fatty substances of the blood, it was found in the early tests of this concept that the average amount of fatty substances in the blood of heart attack survivors was indeed higher than the amount in the blood of those who had not had heart attacks. To some medical investigators the implication of these findings was that elevation in amount of the blood fatty substances is in fact associated with the deposition of fatty substances in the arteries and with the narrowing of the coronary arteries. This implication was derived in the following way: Heart attack victims show higher average amounts of fatty substances in their blood than do those without heart attacks; heart attack victims show more coronary artery fatty deposition and narrowing than those who have not had a heart attack. The probable basis for these two observed relationships is that excessive amounts of fatty substances in the blood are associated with excessive deposition of fatty substances in the artery wall and with excessive coronary artery narrowing. While clarification of the nature of this last implied relationship would still require enormous amounts of work and translation into practical application, it would appear obvious that the findings should have been a basis for intense interest and excitement.

A veritable avalanche of work and progress in understanding heart attacks should have followed almost immediately. Such was not the case, unfortunately, because some skepticism developed to dispute the significance of the findings. The skeptics did not actually challenge the observations that indicated a higher *average* amount of fatty substances in the blood of heart attack victims. They were disturbed, however, by the fact that some of the people who had not had a heart attack had greater amounts of fatty substances in their blood than did *some* of the victims of a heart attack. In other words, they were disturbed by the existence of an overlapping in the amount of the fatty substances between the two groups of persons under study. According to the reasoning of the skeptics one would expect that *all* the heart attack victims should show high amounts of fatty substances and all those who had not yet had a heart attack should have shown low amounts of fatty substances in the blood. Further, they thought that the lowest amounts to be found in heart attack victims should be higher than the highest amounts found in those who had not experienced a heart attack. Probably medical history will rarely record examples of more fallacious thinking than that of these skeptics. The fallacious thinking arose out of at least two major sources: first, a serious lack of understanding of the nature of coronary artery disease; and second, a self-deception in the use of words.

A little consideration of the well-established facts about coronary artery narrowing and heart attacks reveals that, in contrast to the views of the skeptics, an overlapping in the measured amounts of the fatty substances between the heart attack group and the non-heart attack group is precisely *what must be expected*, if the concept of a relationship of blood fatty substances with development of coronary disease is correct. The evidence indicates that high levels of blood fatty substances are required if coronary artery narrowing and heart attacks are to develop. If *none* of the people who are now apparently healthy had these high amounts of fatty substances in the blood, we would not expect any of them to develop heart disease. In this event those who had not yet had a heart attack would never have a heart attack and the problem of heart attacks simply would not exist.

Thus the reasoning of the skeptics reduces itself to the manifestly absurd conclusion that heart attacks represent no problem, which, if true, would end our discussion at this point. Amazingly enough, this type of reasoning (which leads to an absurdly impossible conclusion) did not die with its originators many years ago; it can be found in a variety of forms in the medical literature concerning coronary heart disease even today.

The second basis of such fallacious thinking was stated above to have arisen out of a self-deception in the use of words. The particular word involved is *normal*. When a group of persons who have not yet had any signs of a heart attack is studied, many investigators refer to such a group as representing "normals." If they mean by this that such a group is representative of the *apparently* healthy individuals in the population, one could not object. However, a further connotation has been introduced—that if a group of persons who have not had heart attacks are "normals," then they must be free of any coronary arterial narrowing. Since they are free of coronary arterial narrowing, one would not expect to find any of them with high amounts of fatty substances in the blood. Thus, since some of the "normals" *do* show high amounts of the fatty substances in the blood, the *false* conclusion is drawn that fatty substances in the blood cannot be related to the development of coronary artery hardening and narrowing. The error here is in the wholly incorrect reasoning that "normals" are free of coronary arterial disease. It is well known that the arteries of many people who have not yet had a heart attack are quite well advanced in the disease process. Indeed, these are precisely the individuals with a high risk of future heart attacks. Since it is impossible to know who has excessive coronary artery narrowing and who does not among those not yet having had a heart attack, it would be quite impossible by usual examination procedures to have ever produced a group of "normals" free of coronary arterial disease. Thus the fact that "normals" show in some cases high amounts of fatty substances in their blood does *not* argue against a relationship of fatty substances with the development of arterial disease; it is instead a very strong point in favor of such a relationship. In fact, if some "normals" *didn't* show high amounts of fatty substances in the blood, we could be quite sure that fatty substances in the blood are not related to the development of coronary artery narrowing.

As with many other valid concepts, violent and unreasoned opposition can delay progress for years and decades, although ultimately the concepts come forth again and are accepted for what contribution they really make to solving a problem. This has very definitely been the case in the past five to ten years with respect to the concept of a relationship of the blood fatty substances to arterial narrowing. Several investigators have realized the unsound, fallacious thinking of those who criticized the very much earlier findings and have renewed the attack upon this whole problem vigorously and effectively. The results of such studies have now given us a springboard for major progress forward in our effort to understand the basis for the development of coronary artery narrowing and heart attacks.

There are some important additional reasons why the more recent approaches to a test of the concept of a relationship of the blood fatty substances with coronary artery narrowing have met with more success then the earlier ones, over and above the elimination of absurd reasoning. These have to do with major technical break-throughs in the methodology available to scientists for the study of the blood fatty substances. A quarter of a century ago there did exist some techniques for the study of the blood fatty substances, but what these techniques provided was simply an estimate of the *total* amount of certain of the fatty substances, and even these estimates were crude because of inadequacies in method. During the ensuing years it has become evident that there is an entirely new story concerning the blood fatty substances which has to do less with the *total amount* present in the blood than it does with the actual way in which these fatty substances are transported in the blood stream. This may be illustrated by consideration of one of the very prominent fatty substances of the blood, fat itself. To the chemist, fat represents a specific type of chemical combination and is to be differentiated from a host of substances that are regarded as fatty in character (primarily because they dissolve in such solvents as ether) but which are not chemically defined as fat. For a long time chemists and biochemists had wondered how it is that the blood of humans is able to carry in it relatively large amounts of fat, even though fat and the watery base of blood (the plasma) are known not to mix well. As a result of numerous investigators' work, it has gradually become clear that such a substance as fat itself *does not circulate in the blood as such*. Instead, the fat is hooked up (chemically) with substances known as proteins, which are soluble in the watery base of the blood. There are several different varieties of such combinations that exist in human blood. In fact, not only are fat and protein hooked up in these combinations, but also several other fatty substances of the blood are united into these combinations. The blood fatty substances are thus really combined with each other and with protein substances to form a new class of substances soluble in water.

This new class of substances is designated by the name *lipoproteins* (from *lipid*, which refers to fatty materials, and *pro-*

tein). It is important to note that there is not just one type of lipoprotein in the blood but several types, differing from each other in several respects, such as size of particle and nature of the fatty substances within them. Several methods have been utilized in studying the properties of such lipoprotein particles and in measuring how much of the various types is present in the blood. One method has provided much more detailed and precise information than the others and is now very widely used medically to study the blood lipoproteins. This method utilizes an instrument known as an *ultracentrifuge*, which is the name given to a centrifuge capable of providing tremendous speeds and hence tremendous forces as compared with ordinary centrifuges. For example, in an ultracentrifuge the watery base of the blood (plasma) can be put into tubes that are whirled around at a speed of approximately one thousand times per second and in so doing produce a force of about two hundred and fifty thousand times the force of gravity. Under such tremendous forces the lipoproteins of the watery portion of the blood are made to migrate, and the various types present undergo separation during the course of the centrifugation. By an ingenious system of lenses and a camera an actual photograph can be made of this migration and separation of the various lipoproteins. From this photograph one can tell readily not only *which* kinds of lipoprotein particles are present, but also *how much* of the various kinds is present in a particular sample of blood.

The technical advances of recent years have provided us with a new look at the fatty substances of the blood in demonstrating that they are actually present in the form of the combinations known as lipoproteins. For our problem of coronary artery narrowing and its relationship to the blood fatty substances, this means that there are new problems but also new prospects. The question is now not only "Do people who develop excessive hardening of their coronary arteries have too much of the fatty substances in their blood?" But also, "Which kinds of lipoprotein combinations may be the ones that are important in this regard?" It has been now proved that certain of the lipoprotein combinations are abundant in the blood of persons with excessive coronary artery narrowing and certain others are not. This finding has in great measure solved an early concern of some investigators, for it can now be explained why the total amount of fatty substances may be relatively low in the blood of a heart attack victim. This can occur because even though the total amount of fatty substances is not excessive, certain particular ones (as lipoproteins) may still be quite excessive and cause serious trouble.

With the refined methods now available for measuring the blood fatty substances in the form of lipoproteins by this method of very high speed centrifuging, the problem of studying the relationship with coronary artery narrowing has been approached in a definitive manner. There are many types of the combinations of fatty substances with protein in the blood which we are designating as lipoproteins. Such lipoproteins range in size from those which are very small particles to those (on a relative basis) which are extremely large. Even the extremely large ones are much too small to be seen by the naked eye, or even the eye aided by a powerful light microscope. It has been possible to see these various particles in the past few years by the use of a microscope more powerful than any which utilizes light. The supermicroscope is known as an electron microscope; with it one can take photographs of the lipoproteins (see Figures 1a through 1c). However, taking pictures of the various lipoprotein particles is a more difficult way to measure them than is the procedure of very high speed centrifuging. It turns out, from careful analysis, that only four major groups of lipoprotein particles are more abundant in the blood of persons with coronary heart disease, whereas several other lipoprotein particles do not appear in any way to be associated with heart attacks.

Figure I

ELECTRON-MICROSCOPE PICTURES OF THE LIPOPROTEINS OF HUMAN BLOOD

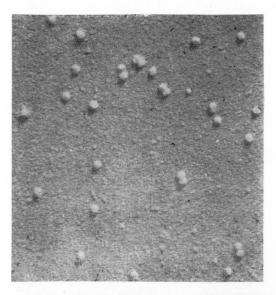

(a)
Lipoproteins of the S_f 6 class, magnified 63,000 times. These are some of the small lipoproteins of human blood. These are part of the group known as the S_f0–12 class of lipoproteins, proved to be associated with human heart attacks.

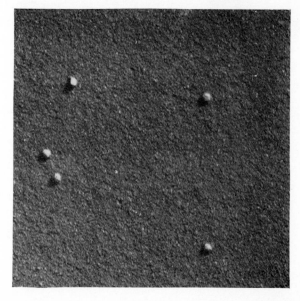

(b)
Lipoproteins of the S_f 13 class, magnified 63,000 times. These are slightly larger in size than the S_f 6 lipoproteins shown in Figure 1a. The S_f 13 lipoproteins are within the S_f 12–20 class, also important for human heart disease.

(over)

Figure I

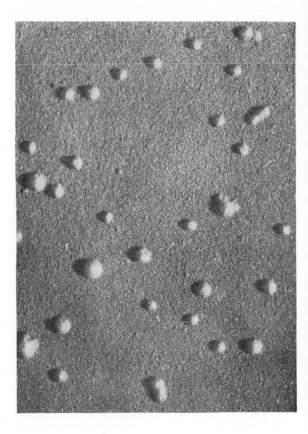

(c)

Lipoproteins of the S_f 17 class and of higher S_f classes in a mixture (magnification is 63,000 times). It is to be noted that many of these lipoproteins are appreciably larger in size than the S_f 6 lipoproteins of Figure 1a or the S_f 13 lipoproteins of Figure 1b. In general, the lipoproteins of higher S_f classes (those which float more rapidly in the superspeed centrifuge) are larger in size than those of lower S_f classes. The lipoproteins shown here are also involved in human coronary heart attacks.

It would be much beyond the scope of this book to describe in great detail the technical aspects of the measurement of the various lipoprotein particles. The principles involved, however, are very simple and deserve mention here. Especially is this important because all of our concepts of prevention of heart attacks (to be discussed in Chapter 14) are dependent upon knowing which of the four important groups of lipoproteins are high in amount in the blood of a particular person.

As stated above, the lipoproteins are measured by their rate of movement in a powerful centrifuge. Since under the conditions of measurement the lipoproteins are lighter (less dense) than the liquid in which they are dissolved, they float to the surface of the liquid under the influence of the powerful centrifugal force, as would cream in a cream separator. What we measure from the photographs of their movement is how much lipoprotein is present at every flotation speed. The unit of speed under such conditions in the centrifuge is known as the S_f unit. In this term the little f stands for flotation, since the lipoprotein particles do float, and the S is a term for the speed, named in honor of the great Swedish chemist Svedberg, who designed the type of centrifuge which makes such studies possible. If a lipoprotein particle floats with a speed of 10 units in this high speed centrifuge, the particle is said to be a lipoprotein of the S_f 10 class, or group. Similarly, if it floats with a speed of 20 units, it is named a lipoprotein of the S_f 20 class, and so on for any speed. The actual measurements are made for several groupings of speeds in the centrifuge. Thus we refer to those lipoproteins that float with speeds less than 12 S_f units as the S_f 0–12 lipoprotein class, those which float with speeds between 12 and 20 S_f units as the S_f 12–20 lipoprotein class. It has been proved conclusively, from many many thousands of analyses, that the particular classes of lipoproteins that are excessive in amount in the blood of persons who have suffered a heart attack are the following:

The S$_f$ 0– 12 class
The S$_f$ 12– 20 class
The S$_f$ 20–100 class
The S$_f$ 100–400 class

Each of these lipoprotein classes is important, therefore, because of its relationship to excessive hardening of the coronary arteries and to heart attacks. It has been found that the higher amount of lipoproteins in the blood of heart attack sufferers is not uniform for all the cases. Thus one heart attack sufferer may show excessive amounts of the S$_f$ 0–12 lipoproteins as compared with "normal" people, but no excessive amount of S$_f$ 12–20, S$_f$ 20–100, or S$_f$ 100–400 lipoproteins. Another heart attack sufferer may show excessive amounts of S$_f$ 20–100 lipoproteins, but no excessive amount of S$_f$ 0–12, S$_f$ 12–20, or S$_f$ 100–400 lipoproteins. Still others may show some combination of the four lipoprotein groups excessive in amount. The crucial point is that, on the average, all four of these groups of lipoproteins are excessive in amount in the blood of persons who are developing excessive coronary artery hardening and who hence suffer more frequent heart attacks. For purposes of understanding what is the root of a particular person's difficulty, it is essential to know which of the classes of lipoproteins is high in amount. But for other purposes of rating a person with respect to the over-all picture, a value is needed which combines all the four important classes of lipoproteins.

Such a value has been developed and has been called *The Atherogenic Index* value, because of its relationship with the hardening process (*atherosclerosis*) that goes on in the coronary arteries. Thus, while one person may have primarily the S$_f$ 0–12 lipoproteins excessive, he may still have the same combined value, or Atherogenic Index value, as another person who has primarily S$_f$ 20–100 lipoproteins in excessive amount. With respect to heart attacks and coronary artery hardening, the expectation would be that two people of the same age having the same Atherogenic Index value would rate equally, no matter which lipoprotein classes made the Atherogenic Index value high. But how one would try to prevent heart attacks in two such persons would depend upon *which particular classes of lipoproteins* were present in excessive amounts in the blood.

The way in which it was first conclusively proved that the Atherogenic Index value was higher in persons developing excessive hardening of the coronary arteries is of interest and importance. We know that persons who have survived a heart attack do have, on the average, a greater extent of hardening and narrowing of their coronary arteries than persons otherwise comparable (in age, sex) who have never knowingly experienced heart disease. If high values of the lipoproteins and Atherogenic Index value are related to the fatty deposition and coronary artery hardening, it would be expected that a higher average value would be observed in the blood of the heart attack survivors. This was precisely what was found in a conclusive way!

For this study, the blood of over five hundred persons who were survivors of a proved heart attack was examined for content of the various lipoproteins, utilizing the very high speed centrifuges. For comparison, the blood of several thousand persons of the same age and sex groups who had no known heart disease was similarly examined. It was found that the average amount of each of the four classes of lipoproteins (S_f 0–12, S_f 12–20, S_f 20–100, S_f 100–400) and the combined value—the Atherogenic Index—were strikingly higher in the heart attack survivors than in the group of what we refer to as "control" subjects. The Atherogenic Index values (which gives the total rating from the individual lipoprotein measurements) for both groups are given as follows:

Atherogenic Index value in 522 heart attack survivors = 94 units
Atherogenic Index value in 5000 control subjects = 78 units

Difference   16 units

A question scientists immediately ask themselves concerning

such findings is "Could this difference in Atherogenic Index value have arisen purely by chance selection of a particular group of heart attack victims or a particular group of control subjects?" There exist quite formal methods for testing this possibility. If one finds that the observed difference could have arisen by chance sampling of the populations studied more than once in a hundred times, one is inclined to be unconvinced that the findings are definitive enough. However, if this chance is *less* than one in a hundred, the findings are regarded as acceptable enough to go forward with other aspects of the problem. In the case of the elevation of the Atherogenic Index value observed in the heart attack victims, the calculations show that the chance of this observed elevation having arisen merely by sampling is *less than one in a million*. This chance, then, is so remote that for all practical purposes we are justified in considering the findings as virtually certain. For biological and medical purposes we would go ahead in almost any field with far less assurance than these observations provide.

We may now review the status of our knowledge with respect to this aspect of coronary artery hardening and heart attacks, before considering the vast ramifications of the findings with respect to prediction and prevention of heart attacks. Early observations had shown that the narrowed, diseased coronary artery contained depositions of several fatty materials. These fatty materials must come from somewhere; recognizing this, investigators suggested the possibility that the blood which constantly bathes the coronary artery walls might be the source of such fatty materials. To test the concept that excessive amounts of the fatty substances in the blood might be the basis for deposition of fatty materials in the arterial wall, a quantitative comparison has been made of the amount of certain fatty substances in the blood in heart attack victims and persons who have not had a heart attack. When measured in the form of lipoproteins, which represent the true form in which the blood fatty substances circulate, it has been conclusively shown that the amount of certain lipoproteins, and the combined value, the Atherogenic Index, which summarizes the amount of all the important lipoprotein classes, is *distinctly higher* in the heart attack victims, on the average, than in persons, otherwise comparable, without evidence of heart disease. Since the heart attack victims have more coronary artery fatty deposits and more coronary narrowing than the other group, the observed findings have been taken to support the concept that high values of the Atherogenic Index are closely related to excessive deposits of fatty substances in the arteries and to the coronary artery narrowing of which fatty deposits represent a part.

No one could now seriously contest the finding of higher Atherogenic Index values in the blood of heart attack victims than in the blood of those without heart attacks. He could justifiably state that this finding does *not* prove that the fatty depositions and coronary artery narrowing are actually *caused* by the lipoproteins of the blood, even though this is indeed very plausible. But is it necessary at this point to debate the essentially unanswerable question of cause and effect? In the opinion of the author, the answer is definitely "No." A set of valid observations concerning coronary artery hardening and heart attacks has been made. The observations themselves are beyond question or requirement of any further "proof." To insist on interpreting the observations on a cause-and-effect basis would be folly, for the observations *by themselves* cannot possibly allow for answering the cause-and-effect question. The cause-and-effect question cannot possibly be resolved without further information, so that arguments about it represent a useless drain of energy that is much better expended in capitalizing upon the *observations* themselves to further our understanding of heart attacks. It is an interesting fact that while suspicions of a possible cause-and-effect relationship *led* to the study of the blood lipoproteins, once the observations have been made it is of no moment *what* led to the discovery.

Whatever may ultimately turn out to be the sequence of events that leads to coronary artery fatty deposition and to coronary artery narrowing, the observations will still stand solidly to show that persons with heart attacks, whom we know to have excessive coronary artery narrowing, have a higher average blood Atherogenic Index value than do persons without a heart attack, whom we know to have a lesser extent of coronary artery fatty deposition and narrowing. Where will this observation take us with respect to our problem of understanding the nature of coronary artery hardening and heart attacks? Let us return to the quest described earlier in this chapter—that of seeking out a possible common denominator which might bring together several apparently diverse but definite clues concerning heart attacks.

There is now available a measurable quantity, the Atherogenic Index value, which, through the study of heart attack victims, has been shown to be very definitely related to heart attacks in some way. Can the amount of blood lipoproteins expressed as the Atherogenic Index value possibly be the sought-for common denominator which will enable the meshing together of the various clues available that pertain to coronary heart attacks? The remainder of this book will show that this question can be answered in the affirmative, for by bringing the lipoprotein part of the picture into consideration it has now become possible to see the outlines of an integrated understanding of the problem of coronary artery hardening and heart attacks. To date, no inconsistencies have become apparent in the integrated concept of heart attacks which has evolved. In the remaining chapters this concept will be developed in detail, with the various clues being brought together, and consideration will be given to the implications of the over-all concept for the medical effort to reduce the high mortality caused by heart attacks.

CHAPTER 4

Why Heart Attacks Occur More Frequently as Age Increases

The relationship of increasing age (measured chronologically) with increasing severity of coronary artery narrowing and increasing frequency of occurrence of heart attacks was alluded to earlier as one of the major clues to follow up in our efforts to understand coronary heart disease. It is also important to re-emphasize that the superficial approach to the consideration of the factor of age led to the erroneous concept that coronary artery narrowing and heart attacks were inevitable accompaniments of growing old. The inevitability concept is dealt a crushing blow by the simple observations, recorded over and over, that coronary artery narrowing and heart attacks can and do occur in young individuals, even in their twenties and thirties, with what may be regarded as alarming frequency and that coronary artery narrowing of significant degree can be singularly absent in certain persons who are octogenarians. The problem at hand is that of reconciling an average trend (and a most important one) of increasing coronary disease with increasing age with a very large number of exceptions to the average trend.

It is evident that at least one other factor must be considered along with age if the apparent discrepancies are to be resolved. Resolution of these discrepancies may be expected to enhance greatly the understanding of the over-all heart disease process. Let us list the pertinent observations that can be regarded as solidly based and then consider whether the discrepancies can be resolved by bringing in the possible common denominator described in the previous chapter, namely, the amount of certain lipoproteins (fatty materials in combination with proteins) in the blood:

1. Heart attacks due to narrowing of the coronary arteries are very rare in children, but they can and do occur in children, especially in certain families.

2. Coronary artery narrowing becomes more marked, on the average, with increasing age at least to the age of eighty years, starting with a negligible degree in childhood. However, at any age, some people show marked coronary artery narrowing and fatty deposition, others show an intermediate amount, and still others show almost none of the disease.

3. The occurrence rate of heart attacks in the population goes up steadily with the passage of each decade of life, although of course many persons get to the age of seventy or eighty with no obvious evidence of symptoms or signs of heart disease. These facts are best shown from compilations (for men) of the National Office of Vital Statistics:

Age groups	Fatal heart attack rate expressed in deaths per year
0–20 years	Less than 25 per 100,000 persons
20–29 years	Less than 25 per 100,000 persons
30–39 years	50 per 100,000 persons
40–49 years	180 per 100,000 persons
50–59 years	610 per 100,000 persons
60–69 years	1210 per 100,000 persons
70–79 years	2500 per 100,000 persons

The rate of rise of occurrence of fatal heart attacks with increasing age is phenomenal, amounting to a hundredfold increase when we compare seventy-five-year-old men with twenty-five-year-old men. Yet we know that twenty-five-year-old men do indeed have heart attacks, and that many seventy-five-year-old men escape them. If age is a factor of importance, which it obviously is, but is not the only factor, which it just as obviously cannot be, how can the findings in the young and the old individual be reconciled? Some investigators of this problem have taken what may be regarded as a simple but certainly superficial way out of the dilemma. They have said in essence that since age is a major factor in the disease, but that certain people develop the disease at an early age, say twenty-five years, the answer must be that we are dealing with at least two different disease processes. The one disease, they would argue, occurs in young persons, and the other occurs in people well along in years. If one were to follow such logic through to its ultimate conclusion, one would require not just two diseases but actually quite a number, for we might just as well say that the heart attack in twenty-five-year-olds is a different disease from that in thirty-five-year-olds, the heart attack in thirty-five-year-olds is different from that in forty-five-year-olds, and so on up to age one hundred. While this approach might satisfy a worker in the field that he has removed a dilemma by this convenient renaming of one disease as seven or ten diseases, this neither gets the problem nearer solution nor is this answer even remotely consistent with the observed and known facts about coronary artery narrowing and heart attacks.

In terms of the general clinical picture, including the signs, the symptoms, and the life or death of the patient, heart attacks are closely similar processes at age twenty and at age sixty. Every feature could not possibly be expected to be precisely identical, since twenty-year-olds do differ as people in some ways, at least, from sixty-year-olds. Furthermore, the important feature to consider is whether or not the underlying process of coronary arterial narrowing is really different in persons having a heart attack at different ages. Such studies have been performed by pathologists examining arteries from persons who have died of heart attacks at the age of twenty-five and from those who have died of heart attacks in their sixties and seventies. These studies, in published form in scientific journals, have indicated conclusively that there is approximately the same degree of coronary artery narrowing in the average person who suffers a heart attack at age thirty as there is in the average person who suffers a heart attack at age sixty or seventy.

Here, then, is a strong unifying feature of the disease entity that leads to heart attacks at any age—an essentially equivalent degree of coronary arterial narrowing. This finding is not an unexpected one. For if, as all the previous evidence has pointed to strongly, coronary artery narrowing is the major underlying process that leads to the occurrence of heart attacks, the logical expectation would be that, regardless of age, the average degree of coronary artery narrowing would be the same in various groups experiencing heart attacks. This finding argues strongly against the superficial approach of considering that coronary heart disease is a wholly different disease in the young than it is in the old, or a different disease decade by decade in life. The evidence clearly suggests that we are dealing with a *single disease entity* at all ages and that the crucial feature is that heart attacks become highly likely when the degree of coronary artery narrowing becomes sufficient.

It is possible to state with conviction based upon evidence that increasing age does increase the frequency of occurrence of heart attacks and the degree of coronary artery narrowing. Further, the average degree of coronary arterial narrowing is essentially the same in persons having a heart attack at any age. It therefore appears inescapable that the problem at hand is to understand how it happens that *some* young persons, in the twenties for example, can have developed sufficient coronary arterial narrowing to lead to a heart attack. Quite evidently age alone cannot be the reason why a marked degree of coronary artery narrowing has occurred in a twenty-year-old man. One would have been led to this same statement of the problem had consideration been directed toward answering the question of why, at any age (for example, forty years), we are able to find some persons with almost no coronary artery narrowing, others with a moderate degree of narrowing, and some with a very marked degree of narrowing. Age of the entire group is forty years, and hence cannot be the explanation for the varying degrees of coronary artery narrowing found.

The superficial explanation of the dilemma with respect to the age findings—that at each age coronary disease and heart attacks represent a new type of entity—can be rejected. The finding that the average degree of coronary artery narrowing in heart attack victims is approximately the same, regardless of age, is crucial.

What might the factor be that, taken into account together with the age factor, will make sense out of all the observations available to us? What properties must such a factor have in order to make the parts of this puzzle fit together? Such a factor must help explain why there is more coronary artery narrowing with increasing age, on the average, in the population, and hence a greater occurrence rate of heart attacks with increasing age. It must help explain how at any age, for example, twenty-five years, some persons can have enough coronary arterial narrowing to lead them to a fatal heart attack, whereas others have little or none of the arterial narrowing.

Some simple arithmetic considerations suggest that a factor which operates in conjunction with time would meet at least some of the requirements. Thus, if coronary artery narrowing is regarded as an accumulative process over time, it would be expected that a given factor operating over ten years might produce twice as much narrowing of the coronary arteries as that same factor would produce operating over five years. Such reasoning could be extended from the period of birth to one hundred years of age, with the expected result that, for a given level of this factor, there would be a progressive increase in the average degree of coronary artery narrowing with increasing age. This is precisely what is observed in a human population such as that of the United States.

Secondly, if such a factor were considered to operate in conjunction with time, it would readily be understandable that a high level of the factor could produce in twenty-five years of life as much coronary artery narrowing as is produced in seventy-five years if the same factor operated at one-third as high a level. This concept would lead to a very simple first approximation for the development of coronary artery narrowing, expressed as the following elementary equation:

Coronary artery narrowing = some factor multiplied by time.

It follows also that such a factor could not be at exactly the same level in a sample group of persons out of the population who are all at the same age. Since at thirty-five years of age some persons have a severe degree of coronary artery narrowing and others have little or no narrowing, it would have to be true that some persons have a high level of this particular factor operating whereas others have a very low level.

So much for the hypothetical properties which such a factor would have to have in order to explain the various observational features of coronary artery narrowing and heart attacks. Our attention must be turned now to the fact that a factor with precisely the sought-for properties *does exist* in the human population and it can be measured quantitatively! In the previous chapter conclusive evidence was developed that implicated this particular factor in coronary artery narrowing and in heart attacks, although no claim was made or need be made for a cause-and-effect relationship. This factor is represented by the lipoproteins of the blood which have been shown to be in high amounts in heart attack victims compared with those who have not yet had a heart attack.

If the amount of important lipoproteins, expressed as the Atherogenic Index value, is indeed the sought-for factor that explains the age differences with respect to coronary artery narrowing and heart attacks, measurements of the blood lipoproteins in the population should reveal trends which prove that the criteria set up for such a factor are met. Measurements of the blood lipoproteins by the high speed centrifuge technique are now available for many thousands of persons at practically all ages and for both sexes, for those in a state of apparent health and for those with a variety of diseases, especially for coronary heart disease. In the considerations that follow immediately only the male sex will be discussed, since an entire chapter will be devoted to the problem of the difference in coronary heart disease between men and women.

The test of the concept that the sought-for factor might be the amount of the blood lipoproteins can be started with a consideration of the persons who have survived one or more heart attacks. The blood lipoproteins have been measured in groups of men who have had heart attacks between the ages of thirty and thirty-nine years, as well as those who have had heart attacks between the ages of forty and forty-nine, between fifty and fifty-nine, between sixty and sixty-nine, and between seventy and seventy-nine years. Presented below are the directly measured Atherogenic Index values in the heart attack survivors at each of these age intervals:

Age group of heart attack survivors	Atherogenic Index value
30–39 years	110.3 units
40–49 years	98.3 units
50–59 years	91.0 units
60–69 years	87.2 units
70–79 years	80.7 units

It is to be noted that the highest average Atherogenic Index value is found in the youngest group of heart attack survivors and the lowest in the oldest group. This finding is precisely in the direction we should expect, if coronary artery narrowing is related to Atherogenic Index multiplied by time. Heart attack victims at any age are characterized by essentially similar, severe degrees of coronary arterial narrowing. Therefore, it would be anticipated that the average thirty-five-year-old heart attack victim would have required a *higher* Atherogenic Index value to allow the development in a span of thirty-five years of the same approximate degree of coronary arterial narrowing as occurs with a lower Atherogenic Index value in the span of seventy-five years for the seventy-five-year-old heart attack victim. Similar considerations apply for the intervening age groups. Thus the study of heart attack survivors provides an important substantiation of the concept that coronary artery narrowing may be related to the Atherogenic Index value *multiplied by time*. It further is evident that this concept removes any necessity for consideration of coronary heart disease as a different disease at each age span in which it occurs. Indeed, there was never any valid evidence that it is a different disease at different ages. Previously certain difficulties and apparent inconsistencies were manifest in considering the whole group, so that considering the disease a different one at different ages provided an escape or a substitute for real understanding.

This, however, is not the only test of validity that the concept that coronary narrowing is related to *Atherogenic Index multiplied by time* must pass. There is the observation that in the population at large at a specified age (for example, thirty years), some men are almost free of coronary artery narrowing whereas others have moderate advancement of the disease process, and still others have a severe degree of coronary artery narrowing. This would require, for the population at large, in groups of thirty-year-old men that there be some persons with very low Atherogenic Index values, others with moderate values, and some with very high values. Otherwise no explanation would be available for the range of observed involvement of the coronary arteries with the narrowing disease. Since the values for the Atherogenic Index are available for representative United States population samples, a direct check can be made of this point. Tabulated below are the Atherogenic Index values as they are actually distributed in representative samples of the male population for the age groups twenty to thirty-nine years through sixty to sixty-nine years. The tabulations are arranged by dividing the entire population sample in each age group into ten categories, from the 10 per cent with the lowest Atherogenic Index values up to the 10 per cent with the highest Atherogenic Index values.

Tabulation of ranges of Atherogenic Index values in healthy men of several age groups

Population Subgroup	20 to 29 years	30 to 39 years	40 to 49 years	50 to 59 years	60 to 69 years
	Ranges of Atherogenic Index Values (in units)				
Lowest 10%	8 to 36	23 to 43	23 to 48	35 to 48	29 to 45
Second 10%	37 to 41	44 to 49	49 to 55	49 to 58	46 to 55
Third 10%	42 to 46	50 to 55	56 to 61	59 to 62	56 to 58
Fourth 10%	47 to 51	56 to 60	62 to 67	63 to 66	59 to 63
Fifth 10%	52 to 56	61 to 66	68 to 73	67 to 70	64 to 68
Sixth 10%	57 to 60	67 to 70	74 to 78	71 to 79	69 to 76
Seventh 10%	61 to 67	71 to 77	79 to 87	80 to 85	77 to 82
Eighth 10%	68 to 74	78 to 86	88 to 96	86 to 91	83 to 87
Ninth 10%	75 to 86	87 to 97	97 to 108	92 to 102	88 to 98
Highest 10%	87 to 163	98 to 191	109 to 226	103 to 207	99 to 200

Inspection of these tabulated values reveals immediately that at any age there exists a very large difference in Atherogenic Index values for the highest 10 per cent of the men studied as compared with those for the lowest 10 per cent. There is approximately ten times as high an average Atherogenic Index value in the highest 10 per cent as in the lowest 10 per cent. Furthermore, from follow-up studies made on hundreds of men for as long as five years each, it appears that those individuals in the lowest 10 per cent of their age groups with respect to Atherogenic Index value tend to remain in the lowest 10 per cent, those in the middle 10 per cent tend to remain there, and those in the upper 10 per cent tend to remain in the upper 10 per cent. Thus, as a first approximation, supported by these follow-up studies, one can say that in adult life the persons high in Atherogenic Index at one age are by and large high at all ages, and the persons low at one age are by and large low at all ages.

All these facts may now be considered with respect to coronary artery narrowing and the concept that its progression is measured by the Atherogenic Index multiplied by time. At any particular age (see the table above) there is a wide range of Atherogenic Index values. Therefore, since Atherogenic Index multiplied by time appears to be the important factor, one would anticipate that within an age group there would be a wide corresponding range of the degree or severity of coronary artery disease in the form of arterial narrowing. Since the persons with low Atherogenic Index values tend to remain low and the persons with high values to remain high, this expectation of a wide range of coronary artery narrowing would hold at a particular age, no matter whether we consider twenty- to twenty-nine-year-old men, forty- to forty-nine-year-old men, or sixty- to sixty-nine-year-old men. This is exactly what is to be found in the coronary arteries of men in the population. Based upon examination of such arteries, pathologists have shown that at each of the above-mentioned ages a wide range of degree of coronary artery hardening and narrowing is to be found. The concept—that coronary arterial narrowing increases in proportion to the blood lipoproteins (expressed as the Atherogenic Index value) and to the time over which such lipoproteins have existed—has actually been tested in a much more rigorous way than the semiquantitative manner above. Based upon the lipoprotein and Atherogenic Index values to be found in the population of men at each age up to seventy years of age, and multiplying each Atherogenic Index value by the length of time in years that such a value has existed, it is possible to construct a table which will predict the *average* degree of coronary artery narrowing that *should* exist in the population of United States men at each age up to the age of seventy. This can be compared with actual measurements of the average degree of coronary artery narrowing observed by pathologists in the study of representative material obtained, for example, from individuals who had died of accidental causes. The *predicted* and the *observed* degree of coronary arterial narrowing are presented side by side below for comparison:

Men, age group	Predicted degree of coronary arterial disease	Observed degree of coronary arterial disease
20–29 years	0.2	0.2
30–39 years	0.29	0.33
40–49 years	0.40	0.47
50–59 years	0.51	0.65
60–69 years	0.63	0.80

The general agreement between the *predicted* average degree of coronary disease and the *observed* average degree can be regarded as excellent and as strongly supportive of the concept that arterial narrowing does proceed in proportion to the Atherogenic Index value and to the time over which such values exist. No doubt there will have to be certain refinements of this concept in its present extremely simple form, but it appears quite clear that the basic features and the major outlines of the concept are in good agreement with what is actually observed with respect to coronary artery disease.

What about the heart attack rate increasing with increasing age? Can this also be predicted from the concept of coronary artery disease proceeding in proportion to the Atherogenic Index value and to time over which it exists? Qualitatively, it is immediately apparent that an increasing heart attack rate would be predicted with increasing age from this concept. We know that the chance of a heart attack increases as the degree of coronary artery narrowing increases. The concept of the relationship of lipoproteins and time with coronary artery narrowing leads to a prediction of a greater average degree of coronary narrowing and a greater proportion of the population having high degrees of arterial narrowing with increasing age. The expectation would therefore be an increased heart attack rate with increasing age, as is observed. Quantitatively, the increasing frequency of heart attacks with increasing age is also predictable from this concept concerning lipoproteins operating over a period of time. The details of such predictions and how they are arrived at are presented in Chapter 9, "Prediction of the

Risk of Future Heart Attacks," but the results of those methods can be presented here for consideration of the age problem.

Through the concept of a relationship of heart attacks (and coronary narrowing) to lipoprotein levels in the blood and the duration of time over which they operate, it is possible to estimate how much more likely forty-five-year-old men are to have a heart attack than thirty-five-year-old men, and similarly how much more likely fifty-five-year-old men are than forty-five-year-old men, and sixty-five-year-old men than fifty-five-year-olds. These predictions can be compared with vital statistics such as those listed earlier in this chapter (page 34). The predictions and the observed ratios from vital statistics are given side by side below:

	Predicted from lipoproteins (or Atherogenic Index values)	Actually measured from vital statistics
Heart attack rate, 45-year-old men compared with 35-year-old men	3.0 times	3.6 times
Heart attack rate, 55-year-old men compared with 35-year-old men	9.0 times	12.2 times
Heart attack rate, 65-year-old men compared with 35-year-old men	24.0 times	24.2 times

It is seen from these tabulations that, quantitatively as well as qualitatively, the concept that amount of lipoproteins in the blood operating over time is crucial for coronary disease *is* in accord with the known facts concerning the age trends in this disease.

In summary, it appears that chronological age is a major factor in the development of coronary artery narrowing and in increasing the risk of occurrence of heart attacks. However, age does not operate by itself; it is important, rather, as a measure of the time that there has existed an elevated amount of lipoproteins in the blood—and lipoproteins were shown conclusively in the previous chapter to be associated with coronary artery narrowing and heart attacks. When age is considered in this light the apparent paradoxes of certain persons developing heart attacks early in life and others avoiding them even at eighty years of age are readily resolved. Further, it becomes possible to view coronary heart disease as a single entity independent of age, for the contradictions encountered by consideration of age *alone* disappear when age is considered as the time over which lipoprotein levels have operated. This concept that lipoprotein levels (expressed in the Atherogenic Index values) multiplied by time give us a measure of the extent of development of coronary artery narrowing (which in turn sets the stage for heart attacks) has certain implications for our over-all outlook with respect to prospects for prevention of the disease. While this will be considered in detail later, it is worth while anticipating that discussion now. If high lipoprotein levels operating over ten years will produce roughly twice as much coronary artery narrowing as the same levels operating over five years, the significant approach to prevention will almost certainly come *by intercepting this process as early as possible.* By whatever mechanism high lipoprotein levels come to be associated with the development of coronary artery narrowing, it would be important early in life to prevent this mechanism from continuing to operate because once the mechanism has operated for a long period of years, the coronary arteries will, on the average, be considerably narrowed and the risk of a heart attack high. Even if after this long period of years the process could be interrupted or decreased in intensity, the damage already done might be in large measure irreversible (although this needs to be determined). The prospect of prevention of heart attacks would appear to lie in recognizing those individuals who have high levels of the important lipoproteins early in life and, once having recognized them, to try to interrupt the process whereby high lipoprotein levels become associated with excessive coronary artery narrowing.

The concept that coronary artery narrowing is an accumulative process proceeding in proportion to the Atherogenic Index value and to the time over which it is present further suggests that even if the rate at which coronary artery narrowing occurs is slowed down, heart attacks may still occur but at a much later period in life than they now do. While, therefore, the prospect may be that heart attacks will still occur, it is doubtful that anyone would deny that progress had been made if those who now develop the disease at forty-five years of age were to do so at seventy-five years of age instead.

CHAPTER 5

Why Men Are More Likely to Have Heart Attacks than Women

One of the most striking features of coronary heart attacks is the much greater incidence of such attacks in men than in women, especially below the age of sixty-five years. Indeed, so evident is this difference, especially in the age groups under fifty, that physicians view with skepticism the diagnosis of coronary heart attacks in young women. Comments have repeatedly been made that in this regard the male sex is indeed the "weaker sex" and that males must be considered fragile because of their inordinate susceptibility to this major killer, coronary heart disease. The comparative heart attack rates are available from the published United States vital statistics for men and women, reproduced in the following table.

Fatal heart attack rate in United States
(number of persons per 100,000 per year)

Age group	Men	Women
30–39 years	49 per 100,000	11 per 100,000
40–49 years	180 per 100,000	47 per 100,000
50–59 years	610 per 100,000	191 per 100,000
60–69 years	1211 per 100,000	535 per 100,000

It is readily evident from inspection of this table that in their thirties men have about 4.5 times the incidence, or risk, of heart attacks that women do. By the sixties this has dropped to approximately a two-to-one risk. Thereafter the two sexes approach closer and closer to equal incidence of heart attacks. In the late seventies the disease is not far from equal in the two sexes. Such evidence represents a most dramatic set of numbers, showing the enormously greater susceptibility of young men than young women to heart attacks and the *lessening* of the difference between the sexes with increasing age. These are straightforward observations based upon what has been happening in the United States in this century. No proof beyond the vital statistics is required to confirm this male–female difference. Since this difference is a glaring fact, there can be no choice but to reckon with it in any concept or theory concerning the nature and origin of heart attacks. Any concept that neglects this set of facts passes up a crucial clue in the entire picture of what heart disease is really like. Any theory or concept of heart attacks which is in conflict with the well-established observations concerning the differences in attack rates between men and women simply must be incorrect.

What of this clue concerning the sex difference? How does it fit, if at all, with all the other information at our disposal? Is there a common denominator linking this vital part of the evidence with the other parts? In the light of information developed in the past decade, the last question can be answered in the affirmative! A priori, one could reason that any of a multitude of differences that are known to exist between men and women might be at the root of the observed differences in heart attack rate. But to consider as a *first* possibility that some factor is important, wholly separate from the possible common denominators, is a backward way to approach a problem such as this. In the previous chapters it was demonstrated that we do now know a major factor that is related to the development of heart attacks and to narrowing of the coronary arteries by hardening. That is the amount in the blood of an individual of the fatty materials designated as lipoproteins (see page 24). High levels of these lipoproteins in the blood (expressed as the

Atherogenic Index value) are associated with an *acceleration* of the rate of hardening of the arteries. Hence, when the levels have been high over a period of years, narrowing of the arteries by the hardening process is excessive and the risk of a heart attack is high. This factor, the amount of lipoproteins in the blood, has already been proved to be important with respect to heart attacks. Can this factor be the common denominator which also explains the difference in heart attack rates between men and women, or must we look for some additional factor or factors?

This question has been examined carefully and in quantitative terms, with the result that essentially all of the observations of the heart attack susceptibility in men as compared with women can be explained from the Atherogenic Index values. To understand the evidence that has been brought to bear upon this problem, it is necessary to know the Atherogenic Index values for men and women at various ages. Such measurements are now available for many thousands of healthy men and women in every age decade for several major regions of the United States. First, it can be stated that there are only trivial geographic differences, if any, for the average man or woman in the western part of the United States as compared with someone of the same age in the central or eastern part of the United States. Not only is the average value for men and women of each age known, but at every age the range of values is known. Let us recall that two facts are solidly established about heart attacks in men and women:

1. A large difference in susceptibility to heart attacks exists for young adults, the males being much more susceptible than the females.

2. With increasing age, the susceptibility to heart attacks becomes increasingly more even between the sexes, so that by the seventies the susceptibility is nearly the same in women as in men.

What would have to be the general pattern of lipoprotein

levels, or Atherogenic Index values, in men and women of the population at large to explain these facts that demand explanation? First, it would be necessary that the average Atherogenic Index value and the distribution of values encountered in the young women would have to be appreciably lower than the corresponding values for the young men in our population. If this were the case, the rate of accumulation of hardening of the coronary arteries in young women would be slower than in young men. Hence, in the thirties it would be expected that women would, on the average, have accumulated less narrowing of the coronary arteries and therefore show a lesser incidence of heart attacks, which is in accord with observation.

Second, it would be necessary for the difference in average Atherogenic Index value between men and women to become smaller with increasing age, to explain the observation that the susceptibility of women becomes closer to that of men as age increases.

Third, as was pointed out before, in the seventies the susceptibility of both sexes to heart attacks becomes almost equal. If the lipoprotein levels and Atherogenic Index values are to explain this, not only is it necessary for the gap in Atherogenic Index value between men and women to decrease as they both grow older, but also it would require that at some advanced age the value in women should become equal to that in men and then increase above that in men. The reason for this is that if the women show lower Atherogenic Index values in the earlier decades of life, the only way they could "catch up" with the men in heart attack susceptibility is for them to have a period of life in later decades where they show higher values than men.

If one now looks at the blood levels of the lipoprotein classes which have been proved to be associated with the development of coronary artery hardening and with the development of heart attacks, expressed as Atherogenic Index values, one finds that each of these conditions just described is met.

The average Atherogenic Index values in healthy men and women in the United States

Age group	Average Atherogenic Index values	
	Men	Women
20–29 years	59 units	45 units
30–39 years	69 units	51 units
40–49 years	78 units	58 units
50–59 years	76 units	68 units
60–69 years	74 units	84 units

The average Atherogenic Index value is seen to be lower in women than in men in the early decades of adult life (both males and females are low in childhood). Since the rate of development of hardening and narrowing of the coronary arteries is greater the higher the Atherogenic Index value, the men would be expected to be developing more coronary artery hardening and narrowing in the early decades of adult life. It is therefore not surprising that men should have a greater incidence of heart attacks in the age span from thirty to thirty-nine years than do women.

Second, it is to be seen that although both sexes show an increase in their average amount of lipoproteins in the blood and hence an increase in Atherogenic Index values as they get older, the difference between the men and women, on the average, decreases progressively. After forty-five years of age, the average woman's Atherogenic Index is increasing at a faster rate then that of the average man. The result is that by approximately sixty years of age the average Atherogenic Index value is the same in women and men. This fits very well with the fact that although men have many more heart attacks than women in the earlier adult years, progressively the frequency of heart attacks in men and women becomes more nearly equal as both sexes become chronologically older.

Third, we note that after the age of sixty women, on the average, have even higher Atherogenic Index values than men. As a result, it is anticipated that, on the average, women beyond sixty years of age are accumulating new hardening of the coronary arteries at a faster rate than men of equal age and are making up for the average lesser degree of hardening that they had before this age. This is why it is possible for the difference in heart attack rate in men and women to shrink progressively, to the point where the rate is almost equal for both sexes in the eighth decade of life.

Thus it is seen that the major features of the difference in heart attack rates between men and women can be explained by a known factor, the Atherogenic Index, which expresses the quantity of certain lipoproteins in the blood. This same factor, known to be directly associated with heart attacks and coronary artery hardening, was shown in Chapter 4 to be able to explain the increasing heart attack rate for people as age increases. Not only does this factor explain which sex is expected to have more heart attacks at various ages, but also it explains by how much they should differ. If one calculates out the expected difference for heart attack rates for young men compared with those of young women and for older men compared with those for older women from the Atherogenic Index values, an answer is arrived at which as the first approximation is extremely close to observations recorded on page 47. Therefore, in the qualitative sense and in the quantitative sense, the lipoprotein levels and Atherogenic Index levels appear to explain the largest part, if not all, of the difference between men and women in heart attack rates. The original clue concerning the difference in heart attacks between men and women is thus explainable on the basis of a common denominator, the amount of lipoproteins in the blood. We can see further how the common denominators which pertain to the development of heart attacks do weave through all the evidence and do tend to make an integrated single picture of the disease.

It is important to realize that this single common denominator does explain the major differences in heart attack rate between men and women. Otherwise, research workers throughout the world could invest fabulous amounts of effort and time along fruitless directions in the effort to find a basis for the male–female difference in heart attack rate. If this difference in the amount of lipoproteins were not known to explain the difference in heart attack rates between men and women, one could possibly think of a whole variety of other possible explanations and invest a great deal of effort and research to try to test the validity of each such explanation. For example, one earlier concept has been that the actual coronary arteries themselves are structurally different in men than in women and that this accounts for the difference in heart attack rate between the sexes. It was believed that possibly women have a different kind of coronary artery which is less susceptible to the hardening process, at least in early adult life. On the other hand, since we know that the lipoproteins already explain essentially the entire difference in heart attack rate between men and women, it does not appear fruitful to look for such other factors as a difference in the wall of the coronary artery between the sexes. This is not meant to indicate that one should not investigate the wall of the coronary arteries of men and women in the effort to discover if there are any real differences. However, one should not investigate the artery with the hope of finding an explanation for the difference in heart attack rates in men and women, since this is already quite well explained both in direction and in quantitative degree by the lipoprotein–Atherogenic Index factor, which also explains so many other features of coronary heart disease.

In an *immediate* sense, as the direct factor involved in causing a difference in heart attack rate between men and women, the Atherogenic Index values and their trends with age in both sexes very clearly do explain the major differences observed. This does not mean, however, that the problem is wholly solved as a result of this finding. We *do* know why men would be expected to have heart attacks at a greater rate than women, because of their higher amounts of blood lipoproteins. However, what we do not know at this moment is *why* men have higher lipoprotein levels in the young age groups, on the average, than do women. And we do not know why that as age increases women become closer to men in lipoprotein level and Atherogenic Index values, and eventually surpass them. This remains one of the most important subjects for medical research in this field in the present era. No amount of money and research effort directed toward finding the reason for this difference could be too much effort or too much money, because of the major implications which such a discovery would have for the health of our population.

This question is, of course, obviously closely related to another equally important question: why there is a difference at all from one man to another or from one woman to another in the amount of the important lipoproteins which they habitually carry around in their blood. Though we will be able to consider certain factors—in the family history, in the diet, and in other areas—which can alter these lipoproteins from the usual levels, it is still pertinent to ask "Why, if two men are both thirty years of age, both of the same height, same weight, and eat approximately the same diet, does one have a high level every time his blood lipoproteins are measured and the other man always have a low level?" Obviously this question is also very closely related to why men are different from women in lipoprotein levels.

It is understandable that the question of the difference in lipoprotein levels between men and women should excite the interest and imagination of many research workers. Indeed, much experimental work has been done along the lines of raising the question of whether or not something to do with maleness and femaleness itself is the reason for the difference in the lipoprotein levels. It is known from a variety of other types of evidence, for example, that the levels of certain sex hormones of the female type (estrogenic hormones) are much higher in the circulation of women than they are of men. Further, although both men and women manufacture male type sex hormones, the amount of male sex hormone is very much higher in men than in women. The idea has been considered that possibly it is this high level of male hormone in men and the high level of female hormone in women that in some way influences the body metabolism with the result that the amounts of lipoproteins in the blood usually are higher in the men than in the women. Some investigators have actually administered female sex hormones in very large doses to men. When this is done, the lipoprotein levels in the men tend to decrease and to become more nearly like those seen in the relatively young women. This very interesting phenomenon may shed some light on the understanding of the factors controlling the lipoprotein levels in men as compared with those in women.

However, rather obvious drawbacks exist in terms of trying to utilize this approach as a treatment for men in order to lower the amount of lipoproteins in their blood and thus lower the Atherogenic Index value. If one uses the large doses of female sex hormone necessary to lower the lipoprotein levels in men it has been observed that the men may develop certain characteristics which make them more like females. For example, they may develop tenderness and swelling of the breasts and there may be real interference with their sexual function. These facts, of course, limit somewhat the practical use of this observation concerning the effect of administration of female sex hormones to men. The observation itself is nevertheless of extreme interest and of extreme importance. There exist good reasons why one should by no means view the situation as discouraging from the point of view that the only possible way to lower male lipoprotein levels approximately to those encountered in women *would have to be* by converting them to women or nearly to women. The basis for the conviction that other approaches will be possible is the fact that a large number of men in any population studied do have low lipoprotein levels, just as the women do, and there is no evidence that these men are those with female characteristics.

Probably the most worthwhile approach to this problem would be to try to understand how men having high lipoprotein levels and Atherogenic Index values differ from the men with low values. Such knowledge would in all likelihood provide an approach other than the use of female sex hormones to lower lipoprotein levels. Incidentally, the findings concerning the female sex hormone may also help explain why women become more nearly like men and even increase beyond them in lipoprotein level, in later years. It is known that the production of at least some of the estrogenic (female) hormones decreases as women become older, an occurrence that is paralleled by an increase in their lipoprotein levels. It is entirely possible that these two facts are closely related. This whole area of knowledge deserves intensive further investigation to understand the mechanism that is operating.

In summary, it may be said that in young adult life the lipoprotein levels and Atherogenic Index values of women are lower than in men and just about enough lower to account for their lower heart attack rate in this early period of adult life. The lipoprotein levels become equal later in life, an effect sufficient to account for the fact that the difference in heart attack rate between the sexes decreases. Women develop even higher lipoprotein levels than men in later years, so that they finally approach the same heart attack rate that men show. All of these observations represent an important step forward, clearing away one of the major mysteries of coronary heart attacks. It represents a further demonstration that a clue available simply through observation of *who* develops heart disease can of itself lead to scientific work that helps to produce an understandable, integrated concept of coronary artery hardening and its result, heart attacks.

CHAPTER 6

How Overweight Is Related to Heart Attacks

Heart attacks definitely do occur in the very fat, in the moderately overweight, and even in the very thin individuals in our population. It can therefore be stated immediately that heart attacks can hardly, by any stretch of the imagination, be considered to be a disease of the overweight person alone. Yet there is a tremendous amount of pressure from physicians, from heart associations, from the life insurance industry, recommending that individuals avoid overweight, in the effort to prevent prominent degenerative diseases such as coronary heart disease in the form of heart attacks.

In Chapter 2 it was pointed out that overweight is in some way related to heart attacks and that this represents one of the primary clues concerning factors involved in heart attacks. Certainly there is sufficient evidence on this issue from various types of experience to lead us to evaluate the information seriously. Furthermore, if the information that is available to us concerning the partial, but not perfect, relationship of overweight with heart attacks is at all valid, it is essential that we understand how the overweight factor may operate in increasing the risk of heart attacks. Integration of the evidence from all *valid* sources is essential in the task of understanding the nature of heart attacks. We will want to examine whether overweight operates through some *new* mechanism that can be shown to be related to heart attacks or whether it operates through those factors which are already solidly established and understood and which have been described in the discussion of the relationship of certain blood lipoproteins with coronary heart attacks.

First, let us examine the nature of the evidence which links heart attacks with the phenomenon of overweight. Such evidence arises from several sources. There is the long-standing general feeling which has existed among physicians that being overweight contributes very little to good health, especially in the decades of life beyond the third. Generally this feeling has not been documented, but has been sufficiently widespread for us to take serious cognizance of it. We can recall that a couple of hundred years ago Benjamin Franklin made a statement to the effect that he had never seen anyone who had died of starvation but he had seen many who had died from overeating. His words bring up one major, but unpopular, point concerning the phenomenon of overweight. This point is that people *become* overweight, by and large, simply by *overeating*.

For a long time many patients and persons in the population at large have hoped, believed, said, and thought that possibly something other than overeating accounts for overweight in *them*. However, over two decades ago careful scientific studies were done with persons who were overweight under well-controlled circumstances in hospital wards. A measured amount of food was given to the individuals under study each day and a very careful check was made to determine that no other source of food was allowed to enter their room. Under these circumstances all the individuals who had been overweight found that they were losing weight when their food intake was cut down, much to the surprise, and even the chagrin, of many. It is a common thing for overweight individuals to state that they eat practically nothing or that they "eat like a bird," or that they are starving themselves and cannot possibly understand why they are overweight.

This is not to say that everyone who eats precisely the same amount of food will have precisely the same body weight; this is far from the case. Individuals doing heavy labor can eat as much as twice to two and a half times the food eaten by other members of the population and still not be relatively overweight. Lumberjacks represent a case in point. In those who do very heavy labor a very large number of calories can be taken in and be consumed for energy purposes. Nevertheless, if any individual is overweight at a particular food and caloric intake, it can be said without fear of contradiction that if he consistently cuts down his food intake he will lose weight until he finally reaches some new lower weight at that food intake. He will thereafter retain this lowered weight so long as he does not increase his food intake above his needs. This has been very carefully and abundantly confirmed by scientific medicine throughout the world.

There is one other factor involved that may confuse some people a little. It is not completely certain that the same mixture of foods in the diet will increase body weight to the same extent. Indeed, there is some suggestion that perhaps fat and protein in the diet will not increase weight to the same extent as will carbohydrates, even if one takes in the same total number of calories. But it can still be said, for any particular mixture of foodstuffs, that if less food is taken in than is necessary to supply body needs, body weight *will* decrease. It is important to dwell on the concept of overeating as the prime source—and essentially only source—of overweight in order to prepare the way for some of our later considerations of why the overweight person might be expected to have some increased risk of heart attack in comparison to persons who are not overweight. Some of the evidence is also derived from geographic findings and for certain periods in the history of mankind, such as the periods of privation that have occurred during wartime and in postwar eras.

There is considerable evidence to suggest that in populations where the total food intake is low (and hence the total caloric consumption is low) and where overweight is uncommon or rare, that heart attacks are distinctly less frequent than they are in a population such as that of the United States, where overweight is rife. This evidence would be highly incriminating against overweight per se except for the fact that we are here considering populations living in areas widely separated geographically, differing in ethnic origin, or taking diets differing in specific food composition, and with grossly different environmental surroundings. The criticism can justifiably be raised that perhaps one or more of the multitude of other factors in the environment, the culture, or the genetic background of the individuals might really be the major influence determining the differing heart attack rate in such populations, rather than the difference in degree of overweight.

Such criticisms must be seriously evaluated and should make us skeptical of accepting such evidence as clearly indicative of any specific effect of overweight itself without further supportive evidence. The evidence accumulated in countries undergoing severe privation during wartimes, when the caloric intake in foods is extremely reduced, leads to the conclusion that heart attacks do become less frequent than in the same populations during periods of plenty. Certainly, with the lower caloric intake the average body weight of such populations does decrease. This type of evidence is a little more direct since we are dealing with the heart attack rate in the *same kind* of people during one period when they are eating freely and during another period when they are severely deprived of food. Hence, some of the characteristics such as racial features or genetic makeup do not represent an issue, but still there are such questions as the variety of other altered circumstances of the environment that go along with wartime periods. Even this evidence has been viewed with reservation and skepticism in some quarters as indicative that overweight per se is a major factor in the development of heart attacks.

Perhaps the most clear-cut and definitive evidence concerning the relationship of overweight as such to heart attacks are the studies that have been reported by Dr. Louis I. Dublin, statistician for the Metropolitan Life Insurance Company. In those studies people were divided according to their body weights into groups below ideal weight, at ideal weight, or various percentages above ideal weight. His evidence was derived from studies of policyholders of the Metropolitan Life Insurance Company. The records of deaths and causes of death for such persons were readily available, since they were insurance policyholders. It was found by Dublin that when one compares the death rate due to heart attacks, in terms of the number of heart attacks per thousand people per year or on some other similar basis, that the persons who were grossly overweight *definitely* had a higher incidence of heart attacks than did those who were not overweight. The magnitude of this difference in heart attack rate is worth considering. Overweight does not appear to be one of the factors that *enormously* increases the risk of heart attacks, as would an extremely high level of lipoproteins in the blood and a very high Atherogenic Index value. The effect is, rather, a modest increase in heart attack frequency for overweight people compared with those who are not overweight. From the information available to us through the Metropolitan Life Insurance Company statistics it appears that for individuals who are 30 per cent overweight, the average heart attack rate is approximately one and a half times that of the persons who are not overweight. This is not enormous, but it is very definite, readily provable, and highly significant and important. No one has ever brought forth any evidence that would contradict the life insurance statistics which show this approximately 50 per cent increase in heart attack rate in very overweight individuals compared with those of the ideal weight. Before going further with this evidence, it is very important to emphasize that even a 50 per cent increase in the heart attack rate in very overweight individuals still does not mean that everyone who is overweight is going to have a heart attack. Furthermore, it must again be recalled that many persons of ideal weight and even those who are underweight *can* and *do* have heart attacks. It is now pertinent to examine the possible basis for the relationship which does exist between the phenomenon of overweight and the frequency of heart attacks. Does this introduce a new factor into the integrated picture of coronary heart disease, or is the overweight effect related to others already established, such as the lipoprotein effect?

One popular notion about the relationship of overweight to the occurrence of heart disease, popular both in some medical circles and in lay circles, is that which might be referred to as the "excess baggage" concept. The person who is 20 pounds overweight is likened to an individual who is not overweight but who is carrying a suitcase with a 20-pound weight within it wherever he goes, every hour of the day. The theory behind this concept is that the excess baggage which an overweight individual is transporting at all times represents a load or a strain upon the heart. In spite of the popularity of this concept in so many quarters, there is essentially no valid scientific evidence to support the notion that this excess baggage represents a real load or a strain upon the heart. Indeed, the amount of physical work such an individual does in transporting this "heavy suitcase" is in the direction that is regarded by many authorities as being beneficial for the individual with respect to his heart function. Inasmuch as this excess baggage notion is at present simply a popular one without any scientific evidence whatever to support it, it need not be taken seriously as a basis for the excessive heart attack risk in overweight persons.

We may turn to other possible explanations. It has been noted that it has been possible to measure certain classes of fatty materials in the blood known as lipoproteins, and a value derived therefrom known as the Atherogenic Index which, when high, increases the risk of heart disease in the form of heart attacks. The pertinent question to ask, once one is convinced of the correctness of the insurance statistics indicating that heart attacks are more frequent in the overweight, is "Could it be that overweight itself is associated with any elevation in the average amount of these particular lipoprotein substances of the blood?" If overweight is in general associated with some elevation of the lipoproteins in the blood, this would be expected to lead the overweight group, on the average, to a greater risk of heart attacks and hence to a greater heart attack rate. This question can be examined directly from scientific evidence, since measurements have been made of the lipoproteins of the blood and the Atherogenic Index value in thousands of healthy persons of all degrees of underweight and overweight in the population at large. Thus, if we consider, for example, a group such as men in the age bracket of thirty to thirty-nine years, we might divide them into several categories based upon their weight and then examine whether the lipoproteins and Atherogenic Index values are different in those of low weights, those of intermediate weights, and those of high weights. Since one would not expect tall individuals to have the same "normal" or ideal weight as short individuals, it has become customary to describe a term known as the *relative weight* for a person. The relative weight is the person's actual body weight divided by what weight is considered ideal for his height. If someone weighs 130 pounds at a given height, and if the height and weight tables would indicate a weight of 120 pounds to be ideal for him, we would divide 130 by 120 and obtain 1.10. This would indicate that this person has a *relative weight* of 1.10, or that his weight is 10 per cent higher than his ideal weight. If he were at his ideal weight, his relative weight would be 1.00. In this way we can rank everyone in this group of thirty to thirty-nine-year-old men on a relative weight scale. Persons with a relative weight of 0.80 are 20 per cent below ideal weight; persons with a relative weight of 1.20 are 20 per cent above ideal weight for their height. Then the entire population of men in the group studied can be divided into the various categories of relative weight. In the table below are given the average Atherogenic Index values (the combined value for the lipoproteins important for heart disease) for each of the categories of relative weight, from the very low ones to the very high ones.

**Atherogenic Index values and relative weights in healthy
men between 30 and 39 years of age**

Relative weight category	Average Atherogenic Index value
Between 0.80 and 0.90 (men who are between 10 and 20% underweight)	64.6 units
Between 0.90 and 1.00 (men who are between 10% underweight and at ideal weight)	64.6 units
Between 1.00 and 1.10 (men who are between ideal weight and 10% overweight)	69.1 units
Between 1.10 and 1.20 (men who are between 10 and 20% overweight)	75.2 units
Between 1.20 and 1.30 (men who are between 20 and 30% overweight)	79.1 units
Above 1.30 (men who are more than 30% overweight)	82.0 units

It will be noted that as we pass from the individuals of low relative weight (underweight individuals) to those of high relative weight (overweight individuals), the average Atherogenic Index values do indeed increase. This tells us that, on the average, overweight individuals do have a higher amount in the blood of those lipoproteins that are associated with heart attacks and, therefore, it would be expected that they should experience a higher heart attack rate than should underweight individuals. Furthermore, by statistical methods it is possible to figure out whether or not this extent of elevation of the blood lipoproteins and Atherogenic Index values in the 30 per cent overweight individuals would give rise to the approximately 150 per cent increase in heart attack rates that the insurance people have observed for overweight individuals. By such statistical tests it has been demonstrated that the amount of lipoprotein elevation does indeed explain the largest share of this observed increase in heart attack rate among overweight people. This remarkable fact is still another illustration of how a thread of unity is being woven into the over-all concept of the basis for coronary artery hardening and heart attacks. We find that the relationship of overweight to heart attacks is not just an isolated fact; it operates primarily through a factor, the Atherogenic Index value or blood lipoprotein level, which has been demonstrated to explain the increase in frequency of heart attacks with increasing age, to explain the difference between heart attack rates in men and women, and as we shall see later, to explain still other features concerning the occurrence of heart attacks.

While examining this relationship, however, it is pertinent to realize one very important issue: these are *average* findings. They do not imply at all that every overweight individual will have high blood lipoprotein and Atherogenic Index values or that every underweight individual will have low blood lipoprotein and Atherogenic Index values. For example, listed below is the scattering of Atherogenic Index values for twenty-five randomly selected cases of people who are very low in relative weight, twenty-five cases who are at an ideal relative weight, and for twenty-five cases who have a high relative weight.

Examination of these Atherogenic Index values makes it clear that more frequently high values are encountered in overweight persons than in underweight persons. This is in accord with the higher *average* Atherogenic Index values in the overweight. Two other facts are also clear. *Some* overweight persons show *low* Atherogenic Index values and *some* underweight persons show *high* Atherogenic Index values. It would follow that the overweight individual who shows a low Atherogenic Index value, all other features being equivalent, would not be expected to share the increased average risk of heart attacks that overweight people suffer because of the *average* higher value of the Atherogenic Index. Similarly the underweight individual who has a very high Atherogenic Index value would be expected to have a distinctly increased risk of a heart attack in spite of the fact that underweight people on the average have lower risks of heart attacks. The underweight state cannot be counted on to provide protection to this individual against a heart attack because for some reason his blood lipoprotein levels are high, and this is the crucial issue with respect to the risk of future heart attacks.

Demonstration that high and low Atherogenic Index values can occur in underweight, ideal weight, and overweight individuals

Scattering of Atherogenic Index values in 25 randomly selected men who are more than 15% underweight	Scattering of Atherogenic Index values in 25 randomly selected men who are at ideal weight	Scattering of Atherogenic Index values in 25 randomly selected men who are more than 20% overweight
27	35	49
36	39	54
38	43	57
39	45	57
43	45	59
44	50	59
45	54	59
46	57	60
46	58	60
48	60	60
50	61	62
50	63	65
52	64	68
52	65	74
54	68	76
54	69	77
56	69	80
59	69	81
60	71	84
64	72	94
68	77	103
70	82	106
87	91	107
88	96	116
145	98	130

What is an even more important and fascinating problem is why only some people with overweight seem to be affected, so that their lipoproteins and Atherogenic Index values are high, whereas other people who obviously overeat and are therefore overweight can escape the increase in Atherogenic Index values that, on the average, accompany the overweight state. Again, why some of the individuals who are marked underweight do not enjoy the average protection conferred by the underweight state against having high Atherogenic Index values remains unexplained. These questions are part of the much larger problem to which we have alluded before—why the lipoprotein levels and Atherogenic Index values are what they are rather than some other values. This is a key question in human body function and body metabolism that must be resolved in the ultimate evaluation of the factors that lead to heart attacks and to their conquest.

Some of the reasons for the agreements as well as the discrepancies between weight and Atherogenic Index values are understood and will be elaborated in much greater detail in a subsequent chapter on the nature of relationship between diet and lipoprotein and Atherogenic Index values. Anticipating that discussion at this point, it can be stated that in some people certain of the lipoproteins are elevated when they have a greater daily intake of the carbohydrate type of foodstuff, such as sugars, starches, and grains. In other people, different lipoproteins, also important for heart disease, are elevated when they have too high an intake of animal fats and certain related fats in their daily diet. Since the overweight individual is taking in a greater number of calories than he needs, it is highly likely (depending upon his personal choices of foods) that he is either taking in excessive amounts of animal fat or an excessive amount of carbohydrates, or an excessive amount of both groups of foodstuffs. These excessive amounts of animal fat or carbohydrates in the dietary intake of the overweight person will probably explain the greatest part of the effect of the overweight state upon his lipoproteins and Atherogenic Index. Whether there is anything else specific about the overweight state that accounts for some people having high lipoprotein values is not clear, but it has not been demonstrated as yet. Certainly, a large part of the effect rests in the food taken in the form of excessive animal fat or carbohydrates, or of both.

CHAPTER 7

The Relationship of High Blood Pressure to Heart Attacks

In the minds of many people there is considerable confusion concerning the nature of the relationships between high blood pressure, hardening of the coronary arteries, and the occurrence of heart attacks. To some, high blood pressure means the same thing as heart disease and hardening of the arteries. This is not correct. The blood in the arterial system, which is the conduit system leading *from* the heart *to* the various organs supplied with nutrition and oxygen, is under a fairly sizable pressure in order to drive it to the organs being supplied. It is quite evident that if there were no pressure within this conduit—or pipe—system there would be no supply of critical organs with blood, which would be disastrous. However, this arterial system is the seat of what may be called a very serious disorder because in certain persons, and from several possible causes, the pressure in this system becomes inordinately high. The human population is characterized by quite a variation from person to person in the average pressure which is maintained in this arterial conduit system. Thus if one were to measure the blood pressure in a thousand individuals at a specific age (for example, in men at thirty-five years of age) there would be a large range of pressures encountered in the blood arterial system from very low pressures to some that are quite high. In spite of this, the individuals would otherwise be apparently healthy.

How then does it come to be considered that the blood pressure when high may in some way be related to hardening of the coronary arteries and to the occurrence of heart attacks? First of all, as with so many other parts of the evidence in the entire problem of heart attacks, the suggestion that high blood pressure is in some way related to heart attacks comes from the vast mass of clinical experience of physicians throughout the world. These physicians have noted that coronary heart attacks *seem*, at least, to be a more frequent than average occurrence among patients characterized by high blood pressure. When such a situation arises, it is always extremely important to check through the evidence carefully to determine if the impression is correct. More times than not, when such a widespread impression does exist from practical medical experience, it probably has some validity when measured scientifically. If this were the only evidence, however, the story would not be very strong. Now a vast body of evidence emanating from several sources has confirmed this issue by demonstrating conclusively that when the blood pressure is high, the risk of coronary heart attacks is high. Not only is the evidence such that one can say that when the blood pressure is high the heart attack risk is high, but also we now know the probable mechanism by which blood pressure elevation operates to increase the risk of heart attacks. Let us recall that the major basis for increasing the risk of heart attacks is an advanced degree of narrowing of the coronary arteries by the process of hardening (arteriosclerosis or atherosclerosis). The evidence that has been accumulated indicates strongly and quite conclusively that elevation in the blood pressure persistent over a long period of time does indeed accelerate the rate at which the arteries will harden. This means, therefore, that the person who has maintained a high blood pressure for a long period of time will have more narrowing and hardening of the coronary arteries and will therefore be a more likely candidate for heart attacks.

First let us consider the direct test of this concept in animal experiments. Such experiments have been done both in the dog and in the rabbit. If one feeds these animals a certain type of diet, or diet plus special medications, it is possible to increase the amount in their blood of certain lipoproteins. When the blood level of these lipoproteins is elevated for a sufficient period of time, the animals develop a narrowing of the arteries due to hardening that is closely analogous to the similar process that goes on in the human, although this process is not absolutely identical.

In both the rabbit and the dog, experimenters have done the following types of experiments: They have divided series of animals into two groups and fed them the diets and drugs calculated to raise the level of their blood lipoproteins and produce hardening of the arteries. Additionally, high blood pressure was induced in one of the groups of animals by one or more types of operation. Therefore, there were available two groups of animals, two groups of rabbits or two groups of dogs, both of which were getting the same diet and medications and developed the same extent of elevation of the amount of lipoproteins important for arterial narrowing. One group of animals was additionally characterized by high blood pressure; the other was characterized by the absence of high blood pressure. After a period of several months the special diet was stopped, the animals were sacrificed, and their arteries examined for the development of arteriosclerosis or hardening. It was shown conclusively, both in the experiments done in the rabbit and in those done in the dog, that those animals who had not only the lipoprotein elevation *but also the blood pressure elevation* had much more advanced degrees of hardening of the arteries than did those with only the lipoprotein elevation *without* blood pressure elevation. Since both groups had the same degree of lipoprotein elevation, they were entirely comparable in this regard. There was no other conclusion that could be drawn than that the high blood pressure was itself the factor in leading the one group of animals to develop excessive hardening of the arteries.

From observation rather than experimentation we now have *direct* evidence on this same issue in humans. In one chronic disease hospital there was a large group of patients from whom repeated blood pressure measurements were available during their extended stay in the hospital. In those patients who died the coronary arteries were examined carefully postmortem to determine the extent of narrowing and hardening. Since the blood pressure readings for these persons had been available for a period between six months and several years before death, it was possible to plot the value of the blood pressure that they had had while alive against the degree of hardening or narrowing of the coronary arteries observed at postmortem examination. It was found that there existed a definite and striking relationship between the blood pressure during life and the amount of hardening of the coronary arteries observed postmortem. The higher the blood pressure had been, the greater was the degree of coronary artery narrowing. This type of relationship in the human is completely consistent with the findings in the experimental animal studies. The observations in these humans serve to confirm the concept that the high blood pressure operates to increase the rate at which the coronary arteries harden.

Probably the most impressive, clear-cut, and definitive evidence accumulated directly on the subject of heart attacks and high blood pressure is available from studies emanating from the Armed Forces. During World War II there were, of course, very large numbers of young men enrolled in military service. From this large group some 542 died at a relatively young age of a coronary heart attack. All of these were proved by postmortem examination definitely to have had a coronary heart attack. Dr. Wallace M. Yater, investigating the various reasons why this group of young soldiers had developed heart attacks, recorded many features about them, including what their blood pressure had been when they were inducted into the Army.

Also available to Dr. Yater were the blood pressure readings on a large group of men of the same age who had not developed coronary heart disease. Comparison of the average blood pressure in these healthy (non-heart attack) men with the blood pressure in those who did develop heart attacks showed clearly that the average blood pressure was definitely higher in those who went on to have heart attacks than in those who did not. The difference in blood pressure between the group with heart attacks and the group without heart attacks is large enough that it would not occur even once in a hundred times by chance sampling alone. Therefore these findings appear very safe.

Similar types of evidence have now been produced by many additional studies. One of these is a large-scale, long-term study of the population of Framingham, Massachusetts, extending over many years, sponsored by the United States Public Health Service. In this study it has been shown that if the blood pressures are measured in a large group of people and if these people are observed for a period of a few years, those who develop heart attacks out of the original group do have on the average a higher blood pressure when measured than those who do not develop heart attacks. From the observations of individual physicians, from hospitals, and from clinics have also come numerous reports indicating in groups of patients who are being followed that the blood pressure is higher on the average in those who develop heart attacks than in those who do not. The evidence as a whole is overwhelming, coming from so many different sources of information.

Therefore it can now be stated quite clearly and definitely that elevation of the blood pressure, even without any other symptoms or signs of ill health, is itself a factor, and a very important factor, in people which predisposes them to a higher risk of future heart attacks. The studies previously described, both of human arteries examined at postmortem and of the animals with and without high blood pressure, both point to the explanation that the way in which the blood pressure elevation operates is by increasing the rate at which hardening of the coronary arteries develops. The more hardening of the coronary arteries there is, of course, the higher the likelihood is of future heart attacks.

The reader might be tempted to ask how a higher blood pressure might operate to increase the rate of hardening of the coronary arteries. One of the earliest investigators of the problem of hardening of the arteries, over a hundred years ago, developed a very simple concept of how this hardening might go on, and very likely this concept is as close to the truth as any that has yet been developed. This idea was that the fatty materials of the blood, the lipoproteins, represent the source of the fatty materials that become deposited in the hardening of the arteries. It was surmised that the way this deposition goes on is actually by a *filtration* of the lipoproteins from the blood stream directly into the arterial wall, and that this filtration is aided by the pressure of the blood in the artery. If this is the case, as it seems very likely to be, the higher the pressure in the artery and the higher the filtration rate will be of lipoproteins into the arterial wall; this would thus explain a mechanism by which high blood pressure accelerates coronary arterial fatty deposition, hardening, and narrowing.

One interesting side observation which, when properly analyzed, clarifies the over-all concept of coronary heart attacks still further is that which relates to the infrequent occurrence of heart attacks in young women. In Chapter 5 it was pointed out that young women have a much lower heart attack rate than do young men. All other things being equal, the physician will view with skepticism the diagnosis of a heart attack in a young woman simply because such attacks are relatively infrequent. Indeed, it has been stated in many textbooks on heart disease that heart attacks are extremely rare in young women *unless* certain special circumstances exist. Among these circumstances are usually listed (1) the presence of high blood pressure, (2) the presence of diabetes, and (3) the presence of a family history of early heart attacks. The problem of diabetes and the family history of heart attacks we shall return to later, but at the moment we can focus on one factor that has been commonly referred to as being almost a prerequisite for heart attacks in young women, the presence of high blood pressure.

Why should this notion have arisen? Evidence was presented in Chapter 5 to support the concept that young women have fewer heart attacks, on the average, than young men because they have lower amounts in the blood of those various blood lipoproteins which are involved in predisposing to heart attacks. Thus, since the women are to a large extent protected against heart attacks, compared with men, by having had less of the lipoproteins in their blood during the early years of life, one of the ways in which they could still develop enough coronary artery hardening to develop a heart attack is to have some other factor which offsets the protective effect of the lipoproteins being low. It would thus be expected that if some other factor could operate, such as the blood pressure, that tends to raise the risk of heart attacks in a woman compared with a man, even in the face of lower levels of the lipoproteins she could still develop enough coronary artery narrowing to develop a high risk of a heart attack. The blood pressure is that other necessary factor. Therefore it is not surprising that those women in early life who do develop heart attacks show a much more prominent elevation of blood pressure than do the young men with heart attacks. This is because men who develop heart attacks early in life do so not primarily because of high blood pressure but because they have very high lipoprotein values. But for women, with their strong tendency to have low lipoprotein levels and low Atherogenic Index values, it is not surprising that they need to have this other factor, the blood pressure, grossly abnormal to develop heart attacks early in life.

The meaning of the relationship of high blood pressure to increased risk of heart attacks deserves further careful explanation. What has been shown above is that, on the average, the blood pressure is higher in those individuals who go on to develop heart attacks than in those who do not. This does *not* mean that every individual who develops a heart attack has had a high blood pressure. Quite the converse is true, for there are some individuals who develop heart attacks with low blood pressure, some who develop heart attacks with moderate values of the blood pressure, and some who develop heart attacks with high blood pressure. However, what *is* meant is that there will be more people with elevated pressures among those who develop heart attacks than among those who do not.

Even many physicians have been confused by this issue and have tended to indicate that they do not think the blood pressure is important in spite of the mountain of evidence to the contrary, simply because they can point to many patients who develop heart attacks who have moderate blood pressures. Such patients can and do develop heart attacks because they have a marked abnormality of the other factor, an elevated Atherogenic Index value. Thus, the occurrence of heart attacks in people with moderate blood pressure in no way provides any evidence to refute the now well-established observation described above—that the higher the blood pressure the higher the risk of future heart attacks.

Considerations of prevention of heart attacks will be discussed later, but at this point it should be mentioned that if one were going to try to minimize the risk of heart attacks by control of such factors as the blood pressure and the lipoproteins, one must approach the problem with some common sense and good judgment as well. If it is known, as it is, that high blood pressure is related to heart attacks, then individuals who have high blood pressure and who can be treated effectively to reduce the elevated blood pressure undoubtedly should have their blood pressures reduced.

Some may say that if risk of future heart attacks is lowered by lowering blood pressure, why is it not logical to try to reduce blood pressures even further when the pressures are already quite low. Here we must consider carefully that at least a certain pressure must be maintained in the arterial system in order to drive the blood around to the various tissues, and that if the blood pressure is reduced beyond certain low levels, one can produce serious symptoms and illness due to an inadequate supply of blood. This is very much the type of situation that exists in a variety of forms of traumatic shock. Thus, whereas lowering an elevated blood pressure may be beneficial to reduce the risk of heart attacks, one does have to keep in mind that lowering the pressure further when it is already low may not be logical because a train of other events may be initiated that are highly unfavorable.

The elevation of the blood pressure is a major factor in increasing the risk of heart attacks through the mechanism of increasing hardening and narrowing of the coronary arteries. It is of the greatest importance to realize that elevation in blood pressure is a *second* major common denominator in the story of coronary heart attacks. Up to this point in our discussion of heart attacks we have found that various parts of the evidence led back to the blood lipoproteins and Atherogenic Index values as the factors explaining the evidence. Since the blood pressure is quite definitely related to the risk of heart attacks, another question can now be raised: "Is elevated blood pressure itself a result of elevated lipoprotein levels and Atherogenic Index values?"

This question has been carefully examined and the conclusion is that the relationship of elevation in blood pressure to increase in heart attack risk *cannot* be explained by any relationship of elevation of blood pressure to elevation in Atherogenic Index value. Thus, while the effect of sex and age on heart attack risk is readily explainable through the lipoprotein–Atherogenic Index findings, the effect of elevation of blood pressure cannot be so explained. It is for this reason that we are forced to the conclusion that it is necessary to recognize the blood pressure as a *second common denominator* in explaining heart attacks. The first common denominator is the blood lipoprotein–Atherogenic Index value. The higher the blood lipoprotein level and Atherogenic Index values, the higher is the risk of heart attacks. But, for any particular lipoprotein level and Atherogenic Index value, the higher the blood pressure, the higher is the risk of future heart attacks.

In any new situation where we find that heart attacks are relatively frequent, it now is necessary to determine whether either (or both) of these common denominators (the Atherogenic Index and the blood pressure) is responsible, or whether we need to look for still additional factors as possible common denominators in the genesis of heart attacks. It follows further that, since the blood pressure and the lipoproteins operate as independent factors, both predisposing to the risk of a heart attack, we must consider that a person characterized both by high lipoprotein levels and by a high blood pressure—and there are many such—has the highest risk of a future heart attack. A person who is high in blood pressure but low or average in blood lipoprotein level or one who is high in lipoprotein level but average or low in the blood pressure occupies an intermediary position with respect to the risk of a heart attack.

Finally, the persons who are best off in our population with respect to the risk of future heart attacks are those who have low levels of blood pressure and low levels of lipoproteins. From the point of view of preventive medicine, however, it will be shown that knowledge concerning the existence of two independent factors, the blood pressure and the lipoproteins, gives us a twofold attack upon the problem of preventing heart disease. In some individuals who are high both in blood pressure and blood lipoprotein levels, we are medically capable of doing a better job of lowering one than the other. In such a case one would want to do everything possible to lower one of the factors, since that of itself would help reduce the heart attack risk even though one could not in a particular individual succeed in lowering both factors with currently available preventive or treatment methods.

CHAPTER **8**

Why Heart Disease Occurs with High Frequency in Certain Families

That certain families are characterized by a marked predisposition to the development of coronary heart attacks during relatively early years is a concept that has gained wide credence in both medical circles and among the public. It has been remarked in an earlier chapter that some say the best way to avoid coronary disease is to choose one's ancestors wisely.

The nature of the evidence surrounding this popular concept must be examined carefully. First the question must be asked: "Is it true that certain families are inordinately predisposed to develop coronary heart disease?" Secondly: "If it is true, is it that all members of certain families are unusually susceptible to coronary heart attacks?" Thirdly, the question must be raised: "How does this family predisposition come about?" For example, it is entirely possible that the nature of any such association of many heart attacks in members of a single family might be due to some defect that is transmitted in a hereditary fashion from generation to generation through the germ plasm. Alternatively, it is also possible that there is something either about the habits of certain families or the environment in which they live, whatever we may decide to include in "environment," which may account for this inordinate predisposition to heart attacks, assuming such predisposition really exists. And then we must ask what we know or can learn about a possible *basis* for any relationship that is found to exist between family history and coronary heart attacks.

Does any such relationship introduce a new major common denominator into our over-all concept of the basis for heart attacks? Or does any possible association of family history with heart attack susceptibility operate in some way on one of the two major factors that we know to be predisposing factors in the development of heart attacks—the lipoprotein levels in the blood and the blood pressure?

First let us examine the question of whether or not it is really true that heart attacks do occur in certain families with excessive frequency. It is definitely possible to say that for certain very special families there is no doubt whatever that heart attacks occur with great frequency. Families exist for whom the medical history is known for several generations and in which it has been shown that in each generation there is a great tendency for members of the family to die at an early age of a coronary heart attack, for example between the ages of twenty to forty years. In such families for three or four brothers to die before the age of forty of a coronary heart attack and to have this occurrence repeated in several generations is quite distinctive evidence that a family tendency to develop heart attacks at an early age definitely exists. By statistical chance alone (simply by saying "bad breaks"), it would be extremely unusual for this type of pattern to repeat itself so frequently in a given family in several generations. Therefore for such carefully studied families it can be stated that there is very little doubt that a predisposition to development of early and fatal coronary heart attacks exists. In fact, in such families even the female members do not enjoy the usual protection against heart attacks which characterizes young women in the population at large.

But in such families we do have an understanding of the

basis for the premature heart attacks. In these families careful studies of the blood have shown that a high proportion of the members of the family show extreme elevations of one or more of the important blood lipoproteins and hence of the Atherogenic Index. Certain of these families show high levels of S_f 0–12 lipoproteins, others high levels of S_f 20–100, and still others high levels of all lipoproteins from S_f 0 to S_f 400. With such extremely high levels of these lipoproteins known to be associated with acceleration of the development of hardening of the coronary arteries and hence with increase in the risk of heart attacks, it is not at all surprising that the members of such families are inordinately predisposed to the development of early heart attacks. In such families it can furthermore be shown that even the children of members of the family whose lipoprotein levels are very high may already show massive elevations of the same lipoprotein classes at the age of two or three years. Such children below the age of five years may already have as high levels of lipoproteins as their parents, levels far higher than the average for adults in the population at large. For these children there is every reason to estimate from all the evidence at our disposal that their longevity will, on the average, not be great. There exists an extremely high risk in these children of having developed enough hardening of the arteries in their 'teens and twenties to be prime candidates for heart attacks in their twenties, thirties, and forties. The studies of these families enable us to answer at least two questions for these extreme cases. First, careful studies of the distribution of heart attacks in such families and of the abnormality of the blood in the form of a very marked elevation of the blood lipoproteins indicate that a hereditary mechanism transmitted through the genes is at the root of the difficulties. Methods exist in biology for knowing whether the way a particular disease is transmitted fits a hereditary pattern, and in these cases it very definitely does fit. In some way, therefore, the abnormality of metabolism which leads to high values of the lipoproteins in blood of such families is a transmissible trait through the hereditary mechanism of the germ plasm. The premature heart attacks, we can feel extremely certain, are simply an expression of the fact that the members of these families transmit a defect which makes them unable to maintain their lipoproteins at a low level in the blood. The nature of this hereditarily transmitted defective mechanism in the handling of the lipoproteins is not identified as yet, but we can be sure that the high frequency of heart attacks is hereditarily transmitted. The important issue here is the demonstration that the transmission is by the hereditary mechanism rather than by such a mechanism as a common environment of the family members or some common factor for the family such as diet.

Also, these families can teach us something about the second question that was raised: "If it is true that families can be predisposed to heart attacks, are all members of such families predisposed?" Careful study of the fate of large numbers of members of some of these families with excessive amounts of lipoproteins in the blood and a predisposition to heart attacks has shown that certain members in the various generations "escape." They escape the abnormality of the lipoproteins of the blood and they escape the premature occurrence of heart attacks. It is, of course, to be expected that if they do not show the abnormality in the liproproteins of the blood they will escape the high risk of heart attacks, and indeed they do. Thus, even though the family is predisposed to early heart attacks by the mechanism of having very great amounts of lipoprotein in the blood, this cannot be generalized to each member of the family since some of them escape this abnormality in the hereditary transmission and these are not subject to excessive heart disease risk. This is extremely important for the members of such families, since the generalized impression—that a bad family history, even in these special families, means an almost certain development of early heart disease—is erroneous and leads the person to needless worry. If a member of such a family has escaped the transmission of the trait which leads to the very high level of the blood lipoproteins, this person has no reason whatever to feel that he is inordinately predisposed to the development of heart disease simply because of the family history. Some of the members of such families can live to quite a ripe old age free of such diseases as coronary heart attacks simply because they have been fortunate enough to avoid having the high lipoprotein levels. The generalization is therefore false that *all* members of such special families are predisposed to development of early heart attacks.

This type of evidence, pertaining to families characterized by a very marked disturbance of the amount of blood lipoproteins which they habitually carry, represents special evidence concerning familial aspects of heart attacks. It certainly indicates that a family predisposition can exist and that it can be inherited. What does it tell us for the broad mass of the population, not characterized by this very special enormous abnormality of the blood lipoproteins? Does it tell us, for example, anything about the outlook for an individual who has had one parent die of an early heart attack or a brother or sister who has died similarly? There exist many persons who have heard of family predisposition, and when an early heart attack occurs in the family are terribly concerned that this must necessarily mean that they too are going to have such an early heart attack.

To answer questions in this area our attention must be focused on the broad mass of persons, where most of the heart attacks occur, rather than upon special families with highly abnormal lipoprotein levels. It is in this broad mass of the population that we must resolve such questions as "What is the outlook for the person who has a family history of early heart attacks?" If the outlook is poor, we must determine whether in this broad mass of the population there is anything that is transmitted or is otherwise associated with families that creates the predisposition to heart attacks.

There are two major ways in which one can proceed to try to derive these answers. One is to determine directly by a study of individuals who have had a heart attack at a given period of life (for example at thirty, forty, or fifty years of age), what the real nature of the family history is. Is it true that there is always a family history of heart attacks in an individual who himself had a heart attack at a particular age, compared with those persons who have not suffered heart attacks at that age? Or is it true that heart attacks are two, three, four or more times as frequent in the family background of those individuals who have had a heart attack early in life as in that of those who have not? In an inverse way, one could look at the fate of the offspring of persons who have had a heart attack versus the offspring of those who never did have heart disease during life in order to determine how much more frequent heart attacks are in the offspring of those who have had a heart attack than in those who escaped heart disease.

The second approach to this problem would be to examine those factors in a person that we know are directly related to increasing his risk of development of a future heart attack. Are any such factors different in those people who have a family history of heart attacks than in those persons who do not have a family history of such disease? The amount of lipoproteins in the blood and the blood pressure of the individual are two factors that we now definitely know to be associated with the risk of heart attacks in that individual. We must determine, therefore, what the lipoprotein levels are and what the blood pressures are in persons with a family history of heart attacks and compare them with those of persons without this type of family history. Both of these major approaches have now been applied. Let us first consider the evidence bearing on the question of what the family history is like for those persons out of the broad mass of the population who develop premature heart attacks themselves.

In a recent study by Dr. Menard Gertler and Dr. Paul Dudley White of ninety-seven men who had had a heart attack below the age of forty years, interviews were obtained with these persons and with a series of matched control men who had not had a heart attack. For the men who did have heart attacks below the age of forty years it was found that 45 per cent of their parents were still alive at the time of questioning; for the men of the same age without heart disease 59 per cent of the parents were still alive. This suggested that the mortality had been higher among the parents of the patients with coronary heart disease than among the controls. For the heart attack group, of the parents who had died 65 per cent had died of diseases of the heart or blood vessels, whereas for the control group only 46 per cent of the parents who had died had died of such diseases. The fathers of the patients with coronary heart disease showed a larger proportion of deaths due to disease of the coronary arteries (37 per cent) than did the fathers of the control group (18.5 per cent). The evidence in this study was not definitive with respect to the mothers. Of the coronary patients' brothers and sisters, 28 per cent had died of diseases of the heart or blood vessels; of the control group's brothers and sisters only 8 per cent of those who had died had suffered from these disorders. All of this suggests a higher rate of development of heart disease in the relatives of the patients with coronary heart disease than in the relatives of the healthy subjects. These doctors themselves pointed out that such analysis is subject to some type of error since it was only *in retrospect* that patients with coronary heart disease were asked about the medical history of their parents or brothers and sisters. If these patients were unduly concerned about their own heart disease, they might have tended to remember heart disease in their family better or to have influenced their thinking about the cause of death in their parents or relatives as being similar to their own disease. Nevertheless, these items of evidence taken together with others in the medical literature do suggest strongly that there is a familial factor in coronary heart disease for the population at large as well as for the special families described at the beginning of this chapter.

A more direct approach to this question, and one which gets to the actual factors which we do know are associated with the occurrence of coronary heart attacks, is that of studying the family history of persons in the population in relationship to the factors of blood lipoproteins and blood pressure. If the lipoproteins and the blood pressures are studied in a large group of persons in the population (using a reasonable sampling of the population), can it be demonstrated that either or both of these factors may be different for persons with a family history of heart attacks as compared with all other persons in this population? Precisely these questions have been asked and have been answered in a large-scale study. A group of some 850 men were studied with respect to lipoproteins and blood pressure during a regular employment examination. Wholly apart from the lipoprotein and blood pressure analysis, these men were asked to fill out a questionnaire concerning the presence of heart disease in their mother or in their father, and if such disease did exist at what age this had occurred. An analysis was then made of the blood pressure and the lipoprotein results in the people who had recorded death in father or mother of heart disease and compared with all other people in the group under study.

First, with respect to lipoprotein–Atherogenic Index findings, a comparison was made of those men whose fathers had died of heart disease with those men whose fathers had died of any other disease or who were still living at the time of the examination. For the 115 men whose fathers died of heart disease, the average value for the Atherogenic Index was 76.8 units. For all the remaining 735 men of this same age group whose fathers had never had any known heart disease, the average value for the Atherogenic Index was 67.3 units. This is a striking difference in Atherogenic Index value. A statistical test of this difference reveals that so large a difference could have arisen by chance alone less than one time in one thousand. Therefore it can be regarded as demonstrated with very considerable certainty that the blood lipoproteins and Atherogenic Index values are higher, and appreciably so, in those members of the population with a history of a father's death of heart disease than in those individuals who do not have such a history in their fathers.

A similar type of study was made of the death in the mothers. While there was a smaller number of mothers who had died of heart disease, the Atherogenic Index in their sons was again slightly higher than for those men whose mothers did not have a history of heart disease. This particular study of mothers does not encompass sufficient numbers of cases to stand as a separate proof, although the direction of the effect is the same as that for the case of those men whose fathers had died of heart disease. In an entirely similar fashion the blood pressures of those men whose fathers had died of heart disease were compared with blood pressures of the remaining men in the over-all group. It was found that the average blood pressure in those men whose fathers had died of heart disease was 72.5 units, whereas the average blood pressure for the over-all group was 68.5 units. The difference between these two may appear to be a small value, but there is still only one chance in forty that such a difference could have arisen by chance sampling alone. This blood pressure effect is, however, not nearly so large as is the effect of heart disease in the father on the lipoproteins in the sons.

In assessing the real significance of these findings it is important to point out that the true difference that must exist for patients with a history of heart disease in their father versus those without it must be *even larger* than the one reported here. This study was based simply upon the man's statement that his father did or did not die of heart disease. Since individuals do not know accurately the *type* of heart disease that their father may have had, it is quite likely that a number of men who reported their father had died of heart disease may have had the father die of some form of heart disease other than the type we are interested in, or even of some other disease. All such errors in reporting would have tended to diminish the observed differences, but in spite of this a really large difference in Atherogenic Index values was *still* observed. There is no known way in which reporting errors could possibly have increased the observed differences. Hence, it can be stated quite conclusively that in the population at large there *is* virtually certain alteration of one major factor, the lipoproteins in the blood, and probably a small alteration in the blood pressure, both in the direction of an increased risk of heart attacks, if there has been a history of death of the father from heart disease. It would be expected, therefore, that in the population at large a family history of paternal heart disease does indeed mean a higher average risk in the offspring of death of heart disease. These findings make more general the type of findings that were described for the special families where there is a very strong known disorder of the blood lipoproteins and Atherogenic Index that can be inherited.

These findings are *average* findings arising from comparison of a group of 115 men whose fathers did die of heart disease with some 735 men whose fathers did not die of heart disease, and hence the conclusions derived therefrom hold *on the average*. This point concerning the average has important connotations for the reassurance of the person who does have a paternal history of heart disease. Such a person with a history of heart disease in the father *can* have a high value for the lipoproteins in the blood, a moderate value, or even a low value (as many of them do), although there will be a greater occurrence of high values among those whose fathers have died of heart disease than in the group whose fathers have not died of heart disease. It does not follow by any means that everyone whose father has died of heart disease is characterized by the lipoprotein abnormality that would suggest the higher risk of heart attacks in him. Indeed, many such persons have quite low risks of heart disease. On the other hand, there is a greater chance that a person whose father has died of heart disease will have a higher lipoprotein and Atherogenic Index value than the person whose father has not been afflicted with heart disease. This important point must be borne in mind, for it means that the individual whose father has died of heart disease need by no means assume that he carries an increased risk. Rather, he can find out if he carries such an increased risk by knowing whether his own blood lipoproteins have or have not been affected in an unfavorable direction. If the blood level of his lipoproteins is higher than average, then he may be presumed to have to some extent the same type of defect that his father must probably have had and hence carries an increased risk of heart disease. However, if he is among the many who have escaped this particular abnormality, there is no reason to believe that simply the occurrence of a heart attack in his father makes him more likely to have a heart attack than anyone else. Indeed, individuals with a good family history (absence of heart disease) but who have high lipoprotein and Atherogenic Index values would be more likely to have a heart attack than he would. Similar considerations exist for the small difference in the blood pressure between those whose fathers have had a heart attack and those whose fathers have not. If the individual whose father had heart disease escapes the average effect of blood pressure elevation, he need have no concern on this score of an increased risk of heart disease in himself. The mechanism by which the blood lipoprotein level is elevated in offspring of fathers who have had a heart attack is not at all clear. It is clear that they do have higher average lipoprotein values, but whether this arises in the population at large by any sort of hereditary transmission or by some common familial factor in the environment, such as diet, cannot be ascertained at the present moment. This is an issue which deserves intensive further study.

The precise quantitative extent to which a family history of heart disease operates to predispose an individual to heart attacks is not clear. It is, therefore, difficult to say whether the findings of elevated average lipoprotein values and average blood pressures in offspring of fathers with heart disease explain all of the increased predisposition to heart attacks which is presumed to exist. Undoubtedly, a very large part of any such predisposition is explained by these findings and it may well be that this is the *entire* explanation. The testing of any other possibility would require demonstration that such another possibility bears any resemblance to reality. For example, it has been suggested that perhaps the coronary artery vessels in persons with an extensive family history of heart disease are in some way faulty, that perhaps there is an inherited abnormality of the vessels. This concept has never been proved, and there exist no experimental observations known to the author to substantiate it. If such a defect in the arteries themselves does exist, it remains within the realm of speculation for the moment and would require direct observational proof to substantiate it. On the other hand, it can now be regarded as well substantiated that a primary factor associated with familial heart disease is Atherogenic Index elevation in offspring and a secondary factor is a lesser elevation in blood pressure. Determination of whether or not such a family predisposition exists in a particular offspring requires evaluation of the lipoprotein and blood pressure levels in that individual. If the analyses are favorable, there would be no reason whatever for one to be gloomy about the prospects of heart disease in himself simply because of the unfavorable family history of heart disease.

CHAPTER 9

Prediction of the Risk of Future Heart Attacks

The prevention of premature heart attacks in the population of the United States can be regarded as the major medical problem of our era. How may we hope to go about preventing a disease such as this? It was pointed out in the earlier discussion that one of the major features surrounding the occurrence of heart attacks is the suddenness of occurrence in individuals who had considered themselves to be in excellent health up to the moment of the attack. Application of any measures available now or that might be designed in the future to lower the chance of a heart attack, or the *risk* of a heart attack, therefore requires that some means be devised for identifying those persons in need of such preventive measures *well in advance* of the sudden occurrence of a heart attack.

Ideally, the type of information we would like to have would be a knowledge many years in advance of just who is going to have a heart attack and exactly when this is going to occur. Such extremely precise foresight does not appear at the present time to be within the scope of our knowledge, and it is doubtful that it will be in the early foreseeable future. On the other hand, a tremendous amount of information is at our disposal at this time which would enable us to take large steps toward this ideal goal.

Thus, while it is not possible to state for an individual that in a given number of days, weeks, months, or years he will definitely have a heart attack, it is possible, with information already at our disposal, to state that one individual may be much less likely, say one-third as likely, as the average to develop a heart attack in some specified time period. Some other individuals possess an average risk of developing a heart attack. For certain other individuals it can be stated that they may be two, five, ten, twenty, or fifty times as likely as the average person to develop a heart attack in some such specified time period as one year, five years, or ten years.

Once having characterized persons in terms of their relative risk of having a heart attack in the future, it is possible to apply preventive medical measures for heart attacks just as they are applied in so many medical areas with which we are already familiar. Thus, if measures are known, or are being developed (or will be developed in the future) which would reduce the risk for someone who carries an inordinate risk of future heart disease, it would be pertinent to identify those persons who carry such a high risk so that such measures can be utilized. In this way a *preventive hygiene* would be recommended to those persons who carry an extra risk of developing a heart attack in the future.

Similarly, those persons who are known to show less than the average risk of future heart disease could be told to forget about the problem, since heart attacks are not likely to occur in them. In essence, this would all mean treatment in a preventive sense of a risk of future heart disease, instead of treating established heart disease (where treatment is so difficult). For those persons known to have a higher-than-average risk of a heart attack in the future, say two, five, or ten times the average risk, preventive measures might be urgently advised to reduce this risk. It could be stated fairly that the person involved might have escaped having a heart attack even if he had not taken the preventive measures involved. This is no doubt true. On the other hand, a large fraction of the population would view this problem otherwise. Their view would be that if they are carrying an excessive risk of heart disease and if by rather simple, safe measures there is a chance of reducing this risk of future heart disease, they would prefer to adopt the measures advised to reduce their risk even though they might have escaped anyway. Undoubtedly this feeling would be stronger the more excessive the risk they carry. This problem may also be viewed in another light. If the risk for all persons of a future heart attack were cut in half, *even though we do not know specifically* which individuals are going to have the heart attack, the number of persons having a heart attack in any year in the United States would be correspondingly reduced in half. This would be a monumental achievement in medicine. Even if our considerations were limited to those who were known to be at least twice the average in their risk of a future heart attack, we could, by reducing these risks in half, cut down enormously the problem of coronary heart disease. This is true since it is the persons with high risks who comprise such a large proportion of the group that goes on to develop premature heart attacks.

What information is required in the population at large to preselect those individuals with a high risk of future heart disease? The basic information with which to assign a risk of future heart disease to any person is available to us from the material which has already been described in previous chapters in this book. It is simply a matter now of translating this information into risk calculations. Let us first turn our attention to the measurement of the blood lipoproteins summarized in the Atherogenic Index measurement. It has been shown by large-scale studies of thousands of humans that the Atherogenic Index in those individuals who go on to develop a heart attack in a specified time period after study is higher than in the individuals who remain in health in the same time period. An understanding of the determination of the risk that a particular person will have a heart attack in the future by measurement of the lipoprotein–Atherogenic Index is extremely simple, involving the most elementary of arithmetic.

Let us suppose we start out with 10,000 healthy men at the age of forty years and we want to know how some of the men in this group compare with each other in the chance that they will have a heart attack in a period of two years from the present time. Let us suppose (for purposes of explaining the arithmetic) that in a period of approximately two years 100 of these men have a heart attack and that the remaining 9900 do not. Let us suppose further that the lipoprotein–Atherogenic Index measurement had been made at the outset in each of the 10,000 men. From experience with such measurements in over 25,000 individuals, we know for certain there will be some who will be found to show low Atherogenic Index values, some will be found to have intermediate values, and some will be found to have very high values. Not only do we know this, but we know quite precisely how many people will fall into each range of Atherogenic Index values. Listed below is the group of 10,000 divided into ten categories, each containing 1000 men together with the range of Atherogenic Index values encountered in each category, from the lowest to the highest.

How 10,000 healthy men at age 45 years will be distributed when the Atherogenic Index is determined (divided into groups each comprising 1000 men)

Number of men	Range of Atherogenic Index values for each subgroup of 1000 men
1000 (Lowest category)	23 to 48
1000 (2nd category)	49 to 55
1000 (3rd category)	56 to 61
1000 (4th category)	62 to 67
1000 (5th category)	68 to 73
1000 (6th category)	74 to 78
1000 (7th category)	79 to 87
1000 (8th category)	88 to 96
1000 (9th category)	97 to 108
1000 (Highest category)	109 to 226

The critical question to ask is "How many of the 100 heart

attack victims out of this original group of 10,000 healthy men
are going to come from those with high Atherogenic Index
values, from those with intermediate values, and from those
with low values?" This information is also available to us, from
previous studies which determined the Atherogenic Index values that will be encountered in heart attack patients, so we
can now list for the 100 heart attack victims how many of them
will be found with Atherogenic Index values within each of
the ten ranges of values that encompass the entire group of
10,000 men.

**How 100 heart attack victims at age 45–47 years will be distributed
among the various Atherogenic Index ranges**

Category	Range of Atherogenic Index values	Number of heart attack victims in each Atherogenic Index category
Lowest category	23 to 48 units	2
2nd category	49 to 55 units	3
3rd category	56 to 61 units	4
4th category	62 to 67 units	5
5th category	68 to 73 units	7
6th category	74 to 78 units	9
7th category	79 to 87 units	11
8th category	88 to 96 units	14
9th category	97 to 108 units	18
Highest category	109 to 226 units	27

We see that out of 1000 men who have Atherogenic Index
values in the highest group we are going to have twenty-seven
cases of heart attacks. This can be described as a heart attack
rate of 27 per 1000 per two-year period. Now, if we consider
the group of 1000 men in the group with the lowest Atherogenic Index values, we find two cases of heart attacks occurring
out of this group. This is a heart attack rate of 2 per 1000
per two-year period. We now have the heart attack rate for the
1000 men with the lowest range of Atherogenic Index values
and the corresponding heart attack rate for the 1000 men with
the highest range of Atherogenic Index values. Dividing the
second of these two numbers by the first gives the risk of the
high Atherogenic Index group of having a heart attack, com-

pared with the low Atherogenic Index group. It is evident that the 1000 men in the highest Atherogenic Index group have 13.5 times the risk, or are 13.5 times as likely to have a coronary heart attack in the two-year period as the 1000 men in the lowest Atherogenic Index group. By means of one simple blood measurement we are thus able to pick out of a population of healthy men one group of individuals who are more than ten times as likely to have a heart attack as another group.

Now we can go on with this type of simple arithmetic calculation and fill in the heart attack risk for all the intermediate groups in the table. If we consider one of the middle groups (Group 5, with Atherogenic Index values between 68 and 73 units), we note seven men will have a heart attack out of this group, a rate of 7 per 1000 per two-year period. If we compare this with the group of 1000 men lowest in Atherogenic Index value, we see that there are 3.5 times as many heart attacks per 1000 men, so the risk of being in the middle group is 3.5 times as much as the risk of being in the lowest group. Similarly, if we compare this middle group with the highest group we see that the risk of a future heart attack in the highest Atherogenic Index group is $^{27}/_{7}$, or about four times that of the middle group. This type of simple arithmetic and logic can be extended to all the groups and will give us a table ranking all the groups of men with respect to their risk of having a heart attack in a specified time period. For convenience of relating all the groups to each other we can arbitrarily set the risk for the lowest group as equal to 1 unit and then express all the other risks in terms of some number of times the risk of the lowest group. On this basis the group with the highest Atherogenic Index shows a value of 13.5. Proceeding similarly for each Atherogenic Index group, we can construct a table of risk values all compared with the lowest group set at 1.0.

What does this table of relative risk of heart attacks tell us? It tells us that simply by a measurement of the blood made two years in advance of the occurrence of any of the heart attacks we can divide people into ten groups. Members of the

A tabulation of the relative risk of future heart attacks for each Atherogenic Index category when the lowest category's risk is set at 1.0

Category	Range of Atherogenic Index values	Relative risk of future heart attacks
Lowest category	23 to 48 units	1.0
2nd category	49 to 55 units	1.5
3rd category	56 to 61 units	2.0
4th category	62 to 67 units	2.5
5th category	68 to 73 units	3.5
6th category	74 to 78 units	4.5
7th category	79 to 87 units	5.5
8th category	88 to 96 units	7.0
9th category	97 to 108 units	9.0
Highest category	109 to 226 units	13.5

highest group on this scale are going to have more heart attacks in this time interval than will members of any of the lower groups, and we can measure precisely how many more heart attacks. This does not mean that absolutely no members of the the lowest group could ever have a heart attack. Indeed, we have seen that there is expected approximately two heart attacks per thousand for this lowest group in a two-year period. On the other hand, it also does not mean that all members of the highest groups will have a heart attack, but rather that there will be many more of them having a heart attack than members of the low groups. It is precisely this type of information which we need to plan for the prevention of heart attacks. For, without this kind of information, we would never know who the likely candidates are for a heart attack and hence who is in need of medical management with respect to efforts to alter their risk in a more favorable direction.

So far we have only utilized the information from the lipo-protein and Atherogenic Index measurements, representing the first major factor in the development of heart attacks. But we know (see Chapter 7) that there is another major factor that has been proved to be associated with increasing the future likelihood of a heart attack, the average blood pressure that habitually characterizes a person. Let us now do exactly the same thing for the blood pressure measurement as we did for the lipoprotein–Atherogenic Index measurement and simply rank people in terms of their measured blood pressure values. If we divide the original group of 10,000 men into subgroups of 1000 each we have in the following table the ranges of blood pressure that will encompass groups of 1000 each from the lowest pressures to the highest.

How 10,000 healthy men at age 45 years will be distributed according to blood pressure measurements. (Divided into groups each comprising 1000 men)

Number of men	Range of blood pressure values for each subgroup of 1000 men
1000 (Lowest category)	48 to 63 units
1000 (2nd category)	64 to 67 units
1000 (3rd category)	68 to 69 units
1000 (4th category)	70 to 71 units
1000 (5th category)	72 to 74 units
1000 (6th category)	75 to 76 units
1000 (7th category)	77 to 78 units
1000 (8th category)	79 to 80 units
1000 (9th category)	81 to 85 units
1000 (Highest category)	86 to 110 units

We also know the distribution of blood pressures that will occur in the 100 men who go on to have a heart attack. These are listed below according to how many of this 100 fall into the various ranges of blood pressures, corresponding to those for the subgroups of the original 10,000 men in the group.

How 100 heart attack victims will be distributed in the various blood pressure categories

Category	Range of blood pressures	Number of heart attack victims in each category
Lowest category	48 to 63 units	2
2nd category	64 to 67 units	3
3rd category	68 to 69 units	4
4th category	70 to 71 units	5
5th category	72 to 74 units	7
6th category	75 to 76 units	9
7th category	77 to 78 units	12
8th category	79 to 80 units	15
9th category	81 to 85 units	19
Highest category	86 to 110 units	24

If we now compare the highest category with the lowest category we find that there are twenty-four cases of heart attacks occurring in those with the highest blood pressures whereas there are only two cases occurring in those with the lowest blood pressures. In a completely similar manner we may get the risk in any of the intermediate groups, and by setting the risk for the lowest group equal to 1.0 we can construct a table of relative risk for each blood pressure category.

Tabulation of the relative risk of future heart attacks for each blood pressure category when the risk in the lowest category is set at 1.0

Category	Range of blood pressures	Relative risk of future heart attacks
Lowest category	48 to 63 units	1.0
2nd category	64 to 67 units	1.5
3rd category	68 to 69 units	2.0
4th category	70 to 71 units	2.5
5th category	72 to 74 units	3.5
6th category	75 to 76 units	4.5
7th category	77 to 78 units	6.0
8th category	79 to 80 units	7.5
9th category	81 to 85 units	9.5
Highest category	86 to 110 units	12.0

Now we have two separate sets of information (the Atherogenic Index information and the blood pressure information) which give us a ranking of persons with respect to the risk of having a heart attack. If it had been true that the *same* people who occupy the highest 10 per cent of the population with respect to lipoproteins and Atherogenic Index had occupied the highest 10 per cent of the population with respect to blood pressure, and so on through each successively lower 10 per cent, then the blood pressure story would be precisely the same one told by the Atherogenic Index and we would not need both sets of measurements. However, this is far from the case. A person may have a high value of the Atherogenic Index with either a high level of blood pressure, an intermediate level of blood pressure, or a low level of blood pressure. There is practically no relationship between the two measurements themselves and hence they do provide different information.

Let us consider a person who happens to occupy the lowest group on blood pressure measurement and the lowest group on Atherogenic Index. Such people will be readily found. We can arbitrarily set this person on a scale at a risk of having a heart attack equal to 1.0. Now let us consider another person who on the scale of Atherogenic Index falls into the highest 10 per cent of the whole group. From the previous arithmetic we see that on this basis alone he is 13.5 times as likely as the person in the lowest group to have a heart attack in the two-year period following measurements. Let us assume further that he occupies a position on the blood pressure scale in the middle group (5th category); from the arithmetic in the table he has a risk of 3.5 times that of those people in the lowest blood pressure category. He is, from two essentially independent sources, more likely to develop a heart attack than a person in the lowest category both of Atherogenic Index and of blood pressure. The best approximate appraisal of his risk now is not either one alone but the two risks multiplied together. In other words, his risk is 13.5 times 3.5, which gives us 47.3 times the risk of a person in the lowest blood pressure and Atherogenic Index categories. This is the true risk because he is more likely on the one ground and on the other ground, separately, to develop a heart attack. In this way, using the Atherogenic Index risk and the blood pressure risk multiplied together to get a net over-all risk, one can compare and contrast individuals with any blood pressure and any Atherogenic Index value and place them on a combined scale of risk or likelihood of having a heart attack in a future period, such as the two-year period under discussion.

With such information it is now possible to know who the individuals are who are in very urgent need of medical attention with respect to reducing their risk. To be sure, the presence of a high risk does not necessarily mean that an individual is definitely going to have a heart attack in one week, one month, one year, or even twenty years *but* it does mean, for example, if his risk is ten times that of another individual, that for every one out of a hundred of the individuals in the low-risk category who has a heart attack, there will be ten out of a hundred who will have one in the risk category ten times as high. Intelligent persons faced with this type of situation are likely to say "If my risk is high, and even though I may still escape the disease, I would certainly like to lower my risk provided this can be accomplished by safe, sensible hygienic measures." Again, if everyone in the high risk categories were to lower his risk by half, then at any age we would have half as many heart attacks as we now have. Until heart attacks can be completely prevented, such a 50 per cent drop in the mortality from this disease would certainly be highly welcome.

These facts of predictability of heart attacks in advance raise certain questions. First, since the evidence has shown directly that the predictability of heart attacks is at least good some two to three years before its occurrence, one wonders if it is possible to predict similarly such heart disease five, ten, fifteen, or even twenty years in advance of its occurrence? A second question that is closely related to the first is that which asks at what age it first becomes possible to obtain such predictive information. For example, would it be worth while to study the Atherogenic Index in children? If not, when should one start considering the possibility? A third question that comes up is "Who in the population at large should be studied to determine the possibility of an excessive risk of heart disease because of either a high Atherogenic Index or high blood pressure?"

These are all thought-provoking questions and deserve careful answer here. First, let us consider the question of *how long in advance* it may be possible to use such predictive information, with the secure knowledge already that the information is good for at least two or three years in advance of the occurrence of a heart attack. For preventive medical purposes, the sooner we could identify an individual who has an excessive risk of heart disease as a result of his rapid development of narrowing of the coronary arteries, the sooner we can start to intercept this process with measures directed toward prevention. Hence it would be ideal if the predictive value of the blood lipoprotein test or the blood pressure determination existed many years in advance.

It will be noted that in order to do any predicting at all we need to know the Atherogenic Index in the subjects. The basis for prediction rests in the fact that people with high values have a higher risk of such heart attacks in the future than do people with low values. Quite obviously, then, the only point of concern to determine the period of effective advance prediction is whether or not the people with high Atherogenic Index values tend to stay high and those with low values tend to stay low. If the high values stay high and the low values low for a period of five, ten, fifteen, or twenty years, prediction is indeed possible as much as ten, fifteen, or twenty years in advance of the occurrence of heart attacks. Measurements of the lipoproteins and Atherogenic Index have only been made over the past ten years, so that it is not yet possible to say for a particular individual that his level would remain in the same general range for a period longer than this simply because no measurements are available.

However, there is an indirect way of approaching this question, which suggests very definitely that those who are high at a given period in adult life tend to remain high throughout adult life. The indirect evidence which we have that suggests prediction is possible for periods as long as twenty years before the occurrence of a heart attack is as follows: Many persons have been studied with respect to their blood lipoproteins and Atherogenic Index at one period and then studied again one, two, three, or even five years later, some as many as seven or eight years later. If we consider the lipoproteins for such people—for example, at twenty-five years of age, studied again at twenty-eight to thirty years of age; for those whose first study was at thirty and second at thirty-three to thirty-five; and so on up through sixty-five—we find that in the main the persons who ranked high at one of their examinations ranked high at the next examination in terms of the Atherogenic Index value. The persons who rank in the middle of the group tend to remain in the middle of the group. The persons who rank in the lowest part of the group tend to remain in the lowest part of the group. Therefore, since for every age span of adult life from twenty-five to sixty-five years we can prove that persons tend to remain in the same ranking, it follows that any single individual, on the average, would tend to remain in the same ranking throughout his adult life.

There is, then, every reason to believe that the predictability of risk of future heart attacks really extends not only for a period of two to three years before the occurrence of a heart attack but probably for *as long as twenty to forty years of adult life*. The only reason why it is not possible to state the same conclusion for persons well below twenty-five years of age is that not enough blood studies have been done on youngsters and teenagers with follow-up to determine their later values. The Atherogenic Index values are quite low during this early age period and start to rise steeply in the very late 'teens and in the twenties, especially in the male. The real rises occur somewhat later in life in the female. It does appear quite safe to say that beyond the age of twenty-five a man has already identified himself as to whether he is going to be a high lipoprotein carrier or a low one and remains so in general for the rest of his life. Since the risk of future heart attacks is higher the higher the lipoprotein level, one can say that early in life adults have become identified as those who carry a high risk of coronary heart disease in a period two, five, ten, fifteen, and twenty years in the future. Thus there is reason to believe that it is possible to know the risk of persons not only shortly before a heart attack, but a very long time in advance. This means that risk can be determined early enough that something constructive in a preventive sense can be accomplished. This long period in advance of heart disease for which prediction is possible represents a golden opportunity in preventive medicine, for the earlier the process can be intercepted the more the risk can be reduced in the person. The same type of general reasoning would hold for measurements of blood pressures. If elevated blood pressure is found in a person even in the absence of any other features of ill health, the average risk of future heart attack is higher than if the blood pressure is low.

In the discussion above it was stated that *in the main* the people with high Atherogenic Index values tend to retain high values and the people with low levels tend to retain their low values. The inference was made there that perhaps some people might have low values at one period in life, and ten years later might have high values. This deserves some explanation. The reason why in general the persons with high values tend to retain high values is that in general people tend to retain their usual pattern of dietary habits while healthy. Under these circumstances it would be expected that if the lipoprotein–Atherogenic Index values are high by the time the person reaches the age of twenty-five, they will remain high. However, we do find a certain number of individuals who have gone along for years at a particular body weight, for example 140 pounds, and then because of a change of economic status start to eat more, especially of certain types of foods (see Chapter 10) and may gain 30 or 40 pounds over a period of years. Such individuals will, on the average, increase their lipoprotein levels and Atherogenic Index values as a result of this increased food intake and increased degree of overweight. Whereas they may have had Atherogenic Index values in the low ranges at age twenty-five, they may show much higher values at age thirty-five simply because of the fact that they have gained weight and are eating so much more. However, such individuals know that this is the case. This should create no real problem, for if an individual finds that his lipoprotein value is very satisfactory at one period in life and then eats more and gains weight, he can expect that this value may become elevated as a result of his overeating. This type of individual would have to be rechecked again at his higher food intake and greater weight in order to determine where he stands with respect to future risk of heart disease. In the general case, involving an individual who does not change his dietary habits, it would hardly seem necessary in the light of the present facts to recheck him any more than once in three to five years after the age of twenty-five. Of course, the person who starts with a very high Atherogenic Index value would undoubtedly require more frequent rechecks during a program directed toward reduction of his values.

There is one other point that needs special mention. Earlier, special families were described characterized by extremely high blood levels of certain of the important lipoprotein classes and it was pointed out that the metabolic derangement which leads such families to have such very high levels is an inherited tendency. Yet the identity of such families in the population at large is not known. What is most striking about these families is the fact that when the tendency exists on the inherited basis, not only do the adults show this elevation of certain of the lipoproteins in the blood but children as young as three, five, or ten years of age may show the same disorder. It is especially the very youthful members of such families who are of especial concern, since they start at a very early age narrowing and hardening their coronary arteries at an excessive rate, so that when they reach the twenties and thirties they are already highly likely candidates for the occurrence of serious and even fatal coronary heart attacks. It would therefore be extremely important that at the earliest possible moment at least in these families even the children who are characterized by such an abnormality of blood lipoproteins be identified.

This is no small problem in a country like the United States, since as many as .5 per cent to 1 per cent of the children in the nation may be involved. Thus this may not be a problem of just a few children in this country, but something closer to between 100,000 and 500,000 children. They are the most important persons to consider, for they become the prime candidates for coronary heart attacks at an early period of life, when we least like to tolerate the existence of coronary heart attacks.

There is, of course, a way of picking out these children who should be identified as the carriers of a very high risk of future coronary heart attacks. Let us assume that every adult above the age of twenty-five years were to be studied with respect to the lipoprotein content of the blood, which is a highly practical matter now with techniques that have been developed and are available to the public through physicians. It would then be known who the persons with the very high lipoprotein and Atherogenic Index values are, and who therefore might be among those who have such high values on the basis of a familial, hereditary disorder. *Their* children at any age, even three to five years, deserve immediate evaluation to determine whether they have inherited this disorder and already show the high lipoprotein levels which might be in need of correction. Even as an intermediate step, before everyone in the country above the age of twenty-five has had his lipoproteins evaluated, one could certainly advocate a modified measure. In any family where there has been a known history of abnormal blood lipoproteins, or a known history of early heart attack in any member of the family—as, for example, before the age of fifty years—it would certainly be important that all members of the family, adult or child, be immediately studied to determine whether an inherited lipoprotein disorder exists.

It cannot be overstressed that the aim of an early determination of the Atherogenic Index is to institute early preventive measures where needed, for the earlier such measures are instituted the greater the benefit that can be anticipated to accrue to the individual. It undoubtedly occurs to the reader at this point that if such predictability of the future risk of coronary heart attacks is possible now by such a simple technique as a blood examination, why is this not being done for everyone in the population? We are accustomed to certain routine procedures, such as chest films to pick up early tuberculosis, or the use of whooping cough vaccine for practically every child in the population, or the mass inoculation of the population for poliomyelitis. The answer to this question is that there generally exists a massive amount of inertia in instituting any such procedure without a lapse of sometimes a quarter or half a century after the definitive proof is available that the procedure would be useful. The only exception to this is when a powerful public-spirited organization decides that something ought to be done about the problem and puts its power behind overcoming the many and subtle sources of inertia that exist. Since the finding that the blood lipoproteins will aid in predicting the risk of future coronary heart attacks has only been solidified through the study of massive groups of humans during the past five years, the history of such medical matters in the past would suggest that it would probably be asking too much to expect broad application so soon.

Among the various forces of inertia is the simple problem of disseminating the information both to the medical profession, so that they will know what the facts really are, and to the members of the public, so that they will be receptive to the physician's efforts to get them to understand these facts. Unfortunately, this task alone takes a certain amount of time unless one has available mass media of communication to transmit the information. It would indeed be unfortunate that a delay of twenty to twenty-five years should characterize this step in preventive medicine as it has characterized and still characterizes so many others. In time, that time depending upon the manner in which the inertia can be overcome, such blood analysis will become a standard routine for all adult members of the population and for those children in whom it is indicated, and preventive measures will begin to be applied. But this will require a considerable reorientation in thinking concerning the problem of heart disease. So much of the thinking about heart disease has been that it is a disease of later years, a disease of aging, an inevitable disease. This has increased the difficulty of reduction of these new findings to simple terms and of explaining that the time to do something about this so-called disease of middle and later years is really *in the early years* when the stage is being set for the ultimate culmination in the form of a heart attack. The concept that preventive medicine will in the future be the medicine of choice for adults as well as for children will take hold at some point.

CHAPTER 10

The Relationship of Diet to Heart Attacks

The general impression that the diet consumed by people has a great deal to do with the danger of heart attacks is based upon information that has been derived from a variety of sources over a long period of years. Some of these suggestions have come from observations of different ethnic groups throughout the world who consume grossly different habitual diets from our own. Others have come from observations of the change in the heart attack rate which occurs in populations subjected to severe privation, for example, during war years when rations are limited. Still others have come from the feeding of special diets to experimental animals. Most recently, evidence has come from rather careful studies of diets in normal, healthy humans in this country.

In the vast mass of information relating to the subject of diet and the occurrence of heart attacks there exist a great deal of loose interpretation, a great deal of false impression, and many false conclusions. Yet, the very mass of the evidence itself suggests that there must be some element of relationship between diet and heart attacks. It is our purpose now to sort out this information to determine its real meaning for heart attacks and to understand how diet operates, if indeed it does play a role, in the development of hardening of the coronary arteries and heart attacks. If diet does operate in some way to determine a person's risk of a heart attack, several major points will have to be covered in order to determine whether or not diet brings in a new factor or set of factors involved in the risk of heart disease over and above those which we have already considered.

The other possibility is that diet operates in some way to affect one of the factors which we have already shown to be solidly linked with the development of hardening of the coronary arteries and heart attacks. It will be recalled that the two factors we have already established as being linked to heart attacks are (1) the level in the blood of certain classes of fatty materials known as lipoproteins and (2) the level of the blood pressure itself. Up to this point every *additional* factor associated with heart disease (from whatever evidence the association came) has been reducible to an understanding of how that new factor affects either the blood lipoproteins or the blood pressure, or both. Diet will need to be examined in precisely this same manner.

The geographic evidence has been along these lines. In certain areas of the world, hardening of the coronary arteries is far less marked than it is in countries such as the United States. In many such areas heart attacks are apparently relatively unusual, although the medical recording system for them is far inferior to that which exists in a society in which medical care is advanced. One of the examples is China, where it has been reported that the occurrence of hardening of the coronary arteries is much less frequent and severe than in the United States. The occurrence of heart attacks is said to be unusual in the Chinese. Another area where similar observations have been made is Okinawa, where Dr. P. E. Steiner found during the 1940–1950 perod that Okinawans showed much less hardening of the coronary arteries than did people in the United States, and a lower heart attack rate.

Still another country where apparently good evidence exists on this point is Ceylon, where it was noted that hardening of the coronary arteries was minimal among the native Ceylonese and that heart attacks were indeed rare, but where it was also noted by Dr. H. Cullumbine, who studied this question, that the incidence of heart attacks increased as one went up the economic scale. He found that the Dutch burghers who lived in Ceylon did not show a very different heart attack rate from that shown by the Dutch in Holland. The same was true about incidence of hardening of the coronary arteries. It was early in the course of studies such as these that the people who recorded the observations began to feel that there might be some relationship between the habitual diet consumed by individuals in these countries and the incidence of hardening of the coronary arteries and occurrence rate of heart attacks.

One feature that appeared to weave prominently through much of the evidence from various countries outside the United States is that the amount of fat, and in particular fat of animal origin, consumed by the individuals in these countries was markedly lower than that consumed in the habitual American diet. This led early to a suspicion that dietary fat, and in particular dietary animal fat, might in some way be involved in increasing the average rate of development of hardening of the coronary arteries and in thus increasing the risk of heart attacks. However, numerous criticisms have been leveled against the evidence, which is derived from a study of the incidence of hardening of the coronary arteries and heart attacks in widely different and separated populations throughout the world. Some of these criticisms are very abundantly justified, others much less justified, since they tend to make light of the evidence altogether. Some of the criticisms deserve mention here. First, in some of the countries where the heart attack rate has been reported to be low and where the diet deviates markedly from our own, the life expectancy in general is known to be much below that of our own country for a variety of reasons, including parasitism and infectious disease. When this is the case, it is easily understandable that other diseases will appear to be far more prominent causes of death than heart disease simply because people are dying at an age, on the average, when heart disease in any country is relatively infrequent. Some fallacious notions can arise in this way. However, in some of the evidence derived geographically it appears clear that, even if one compares fifty-year-old men in those countries with fifty-year-old men in the United States (which is the appropriate type of comparison to make), the heart attack death rate in terms of numbers of attacks per thousand men per year is still considerably lower than in our own country.

Some of the critics are prone to point out that when one compares widely separated areas such as Ceylon or China with the United States there are a multitude of factors, geographic, climatic, and environmental, which in a host of ways might have a major influence on a disease like hardening of the coronary arteries or heart attacks. Such critics feel it is unfair to blame the difference in heart disease incidence on the diet consumed by the people in such countries. However, this criticism, too, is often unjustified. For example, in Ceylon one can say that the climate, the environmental factors, geography, and weather must be precisely the same for the Ceylonese natives and for the Dutch burghers. Yet the Dutch burghers show an incidence of heart attacks described by Cullumbine to be similar to that in their countrymen in Holland, whereas the Ceylonese show a very low incidence of heart disease. The one point he noted was that a considerably different diet is consumed by the Dutch burghers and the Ceylonese, although both were living in the same geographic area.

Still another criticism that has been raised concerns the concept that it is the dietary fat that is the important issue. While it is true that in some of the areas of the world where heart attacks are infrequent the diet does happen to be low in fat, in particular, animal fat, it has been pointed out by critics that the diet is low in many other nutrient features, such as in the total number of calories taken in daily by the average person. Further, the body weight of the average individual varies greatly from that for the average person in the United States. These critics ask why one should single out the dietary fat intake as the crucial factor. This criticism cannot be completely refuted, for in some of the geographic areas under consideration it is certainly true that there are numerous other factors in the diet beyond that of the dietary fat intake which might conceivably influence the development of heart disease.

Still another point of criticism is that the ethnic origin of the individuals in some of these countries is considerably different from that of the peoples of the United States, and that this factor must also be taken into account. At first this criticism would seem valid, but on more careful examination its validity is much weakened since it is now known that such peoples as Japanese in the United States, consuming a diet like that of non-Japanese in this country, show a heart attack rate much closer to that for other inhabitants of the United States than they do for Japanese in Japan, where the average diet differs markedly from our own.

Another major source of the evidence concerning the relationship of diet to heart attack rates is studies reported concerning the incidence of heart disease during periods of privation. Such periods of privation, of course, occurred during and after World Wars I and II in several countries where valid statistical information has been accumulated concerning the incidence of heart attacks before, during, and after such periods of privation. Thus, for example, in Norway the incidence of heart attacks was compared in the years before 1942, from 1942 to 1945, and the following years. It was found that there was a marked drop in the heart attack rate during the period 1942 to 1945. During this interval of time, as a result of conditions imposed upon the Norwegians by the Germans, there was a marked reduction in the dietary intake of certain foods, in particular, fat. Therefore many investigators of this problem have considered that the evidence from a country such as Norway would imply that the dietary deprivation of certain foods, particularly fatty foods, had led to a rather abrupt change in a favorable direction in the heart attack rate.

Some of the critics of this type of information are quick to point out that the consumption of shoe leather probably decreased to about the same extent as did the consumption of dietary fat and have asked why it is that the decrease in heart attack rate was not attributed to the decrease in use of shoe leather. Viewed by itelf, such a criticism might not be regarded as facetious, but there does exist a vast body of other evidence concerning the dietary fat intake and heart attacks that would make it unlikely that one should attribute the Norwegian evidence to shoe leather usage.

In Germany after World War I and World War II, it was found that there was a distinct decrease in heart attack rate coincident with the deprivation of food, in particular, fatty food. Again, in the concentration camps in Germany, while it was noted that there were many diseases rife among the inmates, the incidence of heart attacks was relatively low, again associated with a marked deprivation of food. Quite obviously, one could bring up many other factors that accompany the deprivation of food in countries during and after wartime and argue that some of these other factors might be of equal importance to the food intake in determining the heart attack rate. While some of these criticisms cannot be lightly disregarded, the general pattern from country to country has been that one major factor that stands out in all cases is the relationship of food intake with the incidence of heart attacks.

The upshot of all these claims and counterclaims concerning diet and heart attacks is that such evidence by and of itself is inconclusive. In part such evidence is inconclusive because of a wide variety of possible criticisms that can be leveled at any interpretation of the geographic observations and in part because the information itself is often subject to considerable error. If it is truly correct that certain aspects of the diet in various countries under various conditions had something to do with heart attack rates, our objective could hardly be to consider any of the evidence as definitive or final. Rather, we should regard this evidence as suggestive of some areas worthy of careful investigation. What we must do under such circumstances is understand what diet has to do with heart attack rates in our country under the conditions characteristic of our usual living pattern.

In the last analysis, it is under these conditions that our heart attacks are occurring and it is for life under these conditions that we need clear-cut information concerning a possible role of dietary factors in heart disease. There is, therefore, every reason to study the possible influence of dietary factors upon hardening of the coronary arteries and the occurrence of heart attacks in this country under the conditions which currently prevail. Before considering such studies it is pertinent to review what most investigators have regarded as the mechanism underlying the various geographic and privation relationships of diet, hardening of the coronary arteries, and heart attacks. In the several situations where restricted diet and a low incidence of heart attacks have been linked, it was found that the amount of certain fatty materials in the blood of people living under these conditions was low. Since the evidence is powerful that the amount of certain of the fatty materials in the blood (see Chapter 3) is related to heart attacks, it has been believed that the lowered level of fatty materials in the blood accounts for the lowered heart attack incidence under these conditions. Indeed, in essentially all of the recent careful studies performed on members of the population in our own country this same general view concerning mechanism has also prevailed. Thus most efforts to study the possible effect of diet upon heart attack rate have focused on the issue of what diet does to the amount in the blood of the various fatty materials, previously described as lipoproteins (Chapter 3).

Fortunately, we are now in a position to make rather definitive statements concerning the role of diet in the development of hardening of the coronary arteries and of coronary heart attacks. Carefully controlled studies of the influence of diet upon the amount of the various lipoproteins in blood have been performed and have led to very clear-cut, unequivocal results. An understanding of these definitive results requires a little further detailed consideration of the nature of these blood lipoproteins. This is of importance because the dietary factors that are operative appear to affect certain lipoproteins of the blood in a manner different from the way in which they affect other lipoproteins of the blood.

Secondly, a major discovery has been that whereas certain elements of the diet may affect one class of lipoproteins, other elements of the diet (previously unsuspected) affect *other* classes of blood lipoproteins important in the development of heart attacks. If we now recall briefly the various lipoproteins that exist in the blood, especially those which are implicated in heart disease, we will remember that the lipoproteins occur in the blood in various sizes, from small particles to very large ones. Those that have been implicated in the development of hardening of the coronary arteries and heart attacks are in two major groups, those known as the S_f 0–20 lipoproteins (comprising some of the relatively small lipoproteins in the blood although not the smallest particles) and the S_f 20–400 lipoproteins (comprising those which are considerably larger than the S_f 0–20 class, but still not the largest lipoproteins in the blood). These two major classes of lipoproteins are of distinct importance for the development of heart disease, a fact that has been clearly proved in the human population *in the United States*. If these are the lipoproteins in the blood which are of consequence for heart disease, any effect of diet upon heart disease via its effect upon the blood must be analyzed in terms of the effect of various items of the diet on each of these important lipoprotein classes. Careful experimental observations have been made of the effect of various elements of the diet upon both of these classes of lipoprotein substances.

Such carefully controlled studies of persons in the United States over long periods of time where the diet is successively altered from one composition to another have shown that the amounts of the S_f 0–20 class of lipoproteins in the blood can be raised, on the average, by increasing the dietary intake of animal fats and can be lowered by decreasing the dietary intake of such animal fats. This conclusion was reached from very careful studies of several groups of humans by investigators in widely separated areas. In some of the individuals studied, the extent to which the lipoproteins of the S_f 0–20 class were elevated by an increase in their dietary intake of animal fats was very great, and conversely the extent to which their lipoproteins of this class could be lowered by lowering the intake of dietary animal fat was very great. For other individuals such effects were much smaller or nearly nonexistent. Therefore it is not correct to make the generalization that, for all humans, raising the intake of animal fat will raise the levels of lipoproteins in the blood or, for all humans, that lowering the habitual amount of animal fat consumed would lower these lipoprotein levels. Rather, it is an average finding that the blood level of S_f 0–20 lipoproteins will rise or fall depending upon the animal fat intake, with considerable variation from person to person as to the magnitude of the effect.

One of the most striking findings of this type of investigation in humans of the effect of animal fat in the diet upon the lipoproteins has been the fact that while the S_f 0–20 lipoproteins are markedly affected by the dietary intake of animal fat, the other major group of lipoproteins involved in heart disease, the S_f 20–400 lipoproteins, are hardly affected at all by the dietary intake of animal fat. We shall return to dietary factors that do influence the S_f 20–400 lipoproteins, but for the moment the effect of animal fats upon the S_f 0–20 lipoproteins must be explored further.

In some of the earlier work concerning this effect of fat of animal origin upon the S_f 0–20 lipoproteins it was found that, when vegetable fat was added back to the diet as a replacement for the animal fat, the levels of the lipoproteins in general tended to rise toward the values that had existed when the person was eating the full complement of animal fat. This led early to the use of a diet restricted in fats both of vegetable and animal origin, because it appeared that the vegetable fats had an effect very similar to the animal fats. Thus the diets commonly advised to reduce heart attack risk were essentially diets low in total fat content. More recent discoveries in this field have necessitated some modification of this conclusion. These recent discoveries have also had a considerable favorable influence on the satisfaction afforded by diets that can be employed to achieve a lowering of the levels of the S_f 0–20 lipoproteins for purposes of attempting to prevent heart attacks.

In the original work on the effect of vegetable fats in raising the S_f 0–20 lipoproteins back toward the values that had existed when the person was consuming a high animal-fat diet, the various vegetable fats were not distinguished from each other. In the more recent work the vegetable fats have been divided into two major categories, those which have been called "saturated" vegetable fats and those which have been called "unsaturated" vegetable fats. Or, in terms of their consistency, the division has been in general into those which are the hardened vegetable fats and those which are oily or liquid. Among common examples of the hardened or saturated vegetable fats are such substances as vegetable margarines and the solid vegetable shortenings. Common examples of the liquid or relatively unsaturated oils are such oils as corn oil, cottonseed oil, safflower seed oil, peanut oil, and several other oils which are liquid at the usual temperatures. What has been found is that the solid vegetable fats, or the saturated varieties (generally derived by hydrogenation of oils), behave very much like animal sources of fat in their effect upon the S_f 0–20 lipoproteins. However, the liquid, or unsaturated, vegetable oils do not appear to have this unfavorable influence of raising the blood level of the S_f 0–20 lipoproteins. Thus, if a group of persons who have been consuming a fair amount of animal fat in their diet is placed for a period of weeks, months, or even longer upon a diet restricted in all forms of fat, it is found that their S_f 0–20 lipoprotein levels will, on the average, fall quite drastically to a much lower value. Then if they are allowed to have vegetable oils of the unsaturated variety reintroduced into their diet, even to the point where the total amount of fat they now get is equivalent to that they had previously consumed in the form of animal fat, the S_f 0–20 lipoprotein levels still stay down essentially as low as they would with no fat added back to the diet. In contrast to this, if the fat of vegetable origin added back to the diet is of the hardened, or saturated, variety, the blood levels of the S_f 0–20 lipoproteins rise back toward the values (although not perhaps quite as high) that the individual had had while consuming the same quantity of animal fat.

This explains why in the earliest work the various vegetable fats were all considered to have the unfavorable effect of raising the S_f 0–20 lipoproteins. For, when the vegetable fats were added to the diet, they were added back in a mixed form, including some of the saturated fats and some of the unsaturated ones. But with the more recent findings that the more unsaturated liquid vegetable oils have essentially no effect on the S_f 0–20 lipoprotein levels, it appears that a person can keep his S_f 0–20 lipoprotein levels low by restricting his animal fats and the solid or unsaturated type of vegetable fats while he continues to consume appreciable quantities of the liquid vegetable oils. This makes adherence to a diet restricted in animal fats a considerably easier and more pleasant task because the liquid vegetable oils increase palatability and satiety value of the diet considerably over one low in all forms of fat. The average reader of this book is of course not a chemist and therefore may wonder what is meant by the terms "saturated" and "unsaturated" fat. Since the need is great to differentiate the vegetable fats into the unsaturated fats and the saturated fats, this question of the meaning of "saturated" must be answered here.

A fat is chemically composed of two major constituents in chemical combination. The first of these constituents is an alcohol known as glycerine, the second one or another of a series of chemical substances known as fatty acids. The fatty acids are composed of the elements carbon, hydrogen, and oxygen. They may be thought of as long, chainlike molecules with the carbons linked to each other like a series of box cars. From the sides of the carbon chain are arms attached to hydrogen atoms. When the carbons of this chain in the fatty acids are holding on to as much hydrogen as it is possible for them to hold on to, they are said to be *saturated* with hydrogen. The fatty acids are then known as saturated fatty acids. If this fatty acid is then further hooked together with glycerine to help form the fat itself, the fat is regarded as a saturated fat simply because the carbon atoms of its fatty acids are holding on to all the hydrogen atoms possible for them.

The amount of hydrogen linked to the carbon of the fatty acid is a quantity that varies. Thus the carbon atoms can hold on to their full complement of hydrogen and thus be fully saturated, or they can hold on to some lesser amount of hydrogen and be partially saturated, or they can hold on to still less hydrogen and be much less saturated (or more unsaturated). The vegetable oils, such as corn oil, cottonseed oil, olive oil, sunflower seed oil, safflower seed oil, peanut oil, soya oil, and a variety of others, have much of the carbon in their fatty acids holding on to less than the full amount of hydrogen. Hence we can say that these oils have unsaturated fatty acids within them and are therefore to a large extent unsaturated oils. It so happens that when the carbon atoms of the fatty acids are holding on to less hydrogen than their full complement, the fats which contain such fatty acids will tend to be liquid, or oily, at usual room temperatures. This is the reason we refer to them as liquid oils rather than as solid fats. However, when the carbon atoms are fully saturated with hydrogen, there is a tendency in general for the fat to be solid at room temperature. Thus it can be quite readily understood that liquid oils of vegetable origin can be converted to solid fats (as in the commercial production of solid shortenings) by the process known as *hydrogenation*.

Hydrogenation is simply a chemical process for forcing the carbon atoms to take up more hydrogen than they already have and thus to drive them toward the point of being more fully saturated. When they are in this more fully saturated form, the fats which they comprise tend to be solid at room temperature. One of the liquid oils, coconut oil, is much more saturated than many of the other well-known liquid oils, and this is true in spite of the fact of its liquidity. Interestingly enough, its greater saturation is accompanied by an action upon the blood lipoproteins much more like that of fats of animal origin than of the other liquid vegetable oils.

One other class of fats is common in the diet, the fats which are derived from such marine animals as fish. To a large extent these fats are of the liquid, unsaturated variety and behave with respect to their effect on the S_f 0–20 lipoproteins as do the unsaturated vegetable oils rather than like the solid, saturated animal fats of dairy or meat origin. Thus fish fat, even though it is truly of "animal" origin, really should be classified for purposes of effect upon S_f 0–20 lipoproteins more on the basis of its unsaturated character, and hence like the liquid, unsaturated, vegetable oils. This is the one major exception to the rule that animal sources of fat have the effect of raising the S_f 0–20 lipoprotein levels, since the marine animal fats do not have this effect.

There has been one major controversial issue involved in the researches concerning the effect of various types of saturated and unsaturated fats upon the blood lipoproteins. This is the issue of whether the animal sources of fat, or the saturated fats, have the effect of raising the blood lipoproteins, or whether the liquid vegetable oils, or unsaturated oils, have the effect of lowering the lipoproteins of the blood. This is a question that is of fundamental practical importance in applying all of this information in the dietary approach to lowering the risk of heart disease. If it were true that the vegetable oils provide some beneficial substance capable of lowering the S_f 0–20 lipoproteins, then one could go on eating all the animal fats (or saturated fats) he desires and simply take a supplement of vegetable oil along with them and still achieve a lowering of the S_f 0–20 lipoproteins. On the other hand, if it is really true that the animal fats have the effect of raising the level of the S_f 0–20 lipoproteins, one could not solve the problem in this simple manner. Rather, it would be essential to *restrict* the diet in animal or saturated fat intake but to allow the use of the liquid vegetable oil freely. Many of the research workers in this field and many physicians have been extremely confused by the evidence on this particular issue. At the present time the most definitive evidence on this subject would indicate that there must be something about the animal fats, or saturated fats, which has the effect upon the bodily economy of causing a rise in the S_f 0–20 lipoprotein levels. There is no good evidence, although some scattered possible bits of evidence, which suggests that the vegetable oils have, of themselves, the effect of lowering the S_f 0–20 lipoproteins. Primarily, the evidence indicates that if one removes fat from the diet to produce a low-fat diet the same lipoprotein levels are obtained as if one adds the vegetable oils back to the low fat diet while still restricting the animal fats. If the vegetable oils were truly beneficial, one would have expected that the level of the S_f 0–20 lipoproteins would be much lower when one eats the vegetable oils than when one eats no oil at all. Since this is not the case, it would appear that the best evidence is that the vegetable oils are without any effect and can be used freely as a substitute for animal fats without raising the S_f 0–20 lipoprotein levels. However, one could not anticipate going on using all the animal, or saturated, fats one desires in the diet and achieve any lipoprotein lowering by simply adding a supplement of vegetable oils to this diet.

In the minds of some physicians and some nutritionists almost everything is interpreted in terms of calories and of body weight. Thus some of these physicians and nutritionists have interpreted the effect on lipoproteins achieved by substitution of vegetable oil for animal fat as due to some loss of calories, or loss of weight. This view is completely incorrect. Experimental investigators in trying to elucidate this problem realized that some would confuse the issue of calories with the issue of what type of fat is eaten. Therefore, they specifically made certain during the studies that the individuals consumed the same number of calories at all times, but simply varied the *source* of their fat while allowing the same *total* amount of fat and the same *total* number of calories. Hence the elevation of S_f 0–20 lipoproteins during consumption of animal sources of fat is due to the *kind* of fat used rather than to the amount of fat per se or rather, in any way, than to the number of calories in the diet per se. Calorie restriction will be considered below, but, for the moment, it is important to stress that the differences described between consumption of animal and vegetable fat have nothing whatever to do with the number of calories in the diet.

It was pointed out above that the S_f 0–20 lipoproteins, one of the major groups implicated in heart disease, are affected by the origin, or type, of fat consumed. The S_f 20–400 lipoproteins, during these same controlled experiments, were unaffected by whether the fat was of animal or vegetable origin. We are, of course, just as intensely interested in the factors in the diet which might affect the S_f 20–400 lipoproteins, since they are at least as important for heart disease as are the S_f 0–20 lipoproteins. The striking and rather unexpected observation in the light of knowledge up to this point has been that another major class of foodstuffs is very important in determining what the level of the S_f 20–400 lipoproteins will be. That class of foodstuffs is the great class known as the carbohydrates, which occur in such well-known substances as the sugars, the starches, the grains, and in the vegetables of the diet, such as beans, peas, and other vegetables.

It was found in carefully controlled studies of individuals on various diets that when the carbohydrate intake of the diet is raised, the average level of the S_f 20–400 lipoproteins is raised too. When the amount of carbohydrates in the diet is again reduced, the S_f 20–400 lipoprotein levels fall back to the previous values. Furthermore, many individuals who are characterized habitually by some type of error in their metabolism that makes their S_f 20–400 lipoproteins habitually extremely high will experience a marked reduction in the blood level of these lipoproteins when the carbohydrate intake is lowered. The calories lost through carbohydrate restriction can be regained by use of vegetable oil. The crucial issue is in this instance the removal of some of the carbohydrates from the diet. Exactly how carbohydrates, which are not fatty at all, can have such a profound influence upon the amounts of the fat-containing blood lipoproteins is not at all clear at the present time. We do know that the body is fully capable of converting carbohydrate substances to fatty materials, which may well have something to do with the mechanism by which the carbohydrates do raise the level of the S_f 20–400 lipoproteins. At the present moment, however, this is not supported as the operative mechanism by any solidly established scientific facts. What is solidly established is that the S_f 20–400 lipoprotein levels, on the average, can be raised by increasing the dietary carbohydrate intake and can be lowered by decreasing it.

These same lipoproteins are essentially unaffected, in the average case, by changing from animal to vegetable fats. This information is extremely crucial, for in many individuals the risk of coronary heart disease comes primarily from the S_f 20–400 lipoproteins. For such individuals, any attempt to lower heart attack risk by shifting from animal fat to vegetable fat in the diet would be illogical. There would be no reason whatever to expect any benefits since one would be changing the diet in a manner directed toward affecting the S_f 0–20 lipoproteins, which is not the problem at hand for these persons. For such individuals, the preventive effort would have to be directed toward lowering the carbohydrate intake, which will, on the average, reduce the S_f 20–400 lipoprotein levels. With respect to the effect of carbohydrates on the S_f 20–400 lipoproteins, it is a matter of the *amount* of carbohydrates that is eaten rather than the total number of calories ingested. For example, if one maintains individuals at exactly the same number of calories per day, so that they do not alter their weight in any way, but takes out some of the carbohydrates in their diet and replaces them by vegetable oil, one finds that the S_f 20–400 lipoprotein levels will fall. Achievement of this result of lowering the S_f 20–400 lipoproteins requires neither any alteration in caloric intake nor any alteration in body weight.

In the discussion of overweight and heart attacks (Chapter 6) it was pointed out that the major way in which overweight becomes associated with increased heart attack risk is through the association of overweight with elevation of the blood lipoprotein levels, and hence of the Atherogenic Index values. In some overweight persons this elevation is in the S_f 0–20 lipoprotein levels, in others the elevation is in the S_f 20–400 lipoproteins, and in still others the elevation is in the level of both classes of lipoproteins. The overweight person achieves this state by overeating. In this overeating he (or she) may consume an excess of animal, or saturated, fat or an excess of carbohydrates, or of both types of foodstuffs. If the excess is in animal-fat consumption, the major effect on lipoproteins will be on the S_f 0–20 class. If the excess is in carbohydrate consumption, the major effect on lipoproteins will be on the S_f 20–400 class. When the overweight person loses weight by calorie restriction, there is a reduction generally in animal fat intake, in carbohydrate intake, or in both. It is most likely that the lipoprotein level lowering which such persons experience by correction of overweight is the result of a decreased animal-fat intake or a decreased carbohydrate intake rather than any specific effect of a reduced number of calories in the diet.

CHAPTER 11

Relationship of Cigarette Smoking to Heart Attacks

Physicians have long been in the habit of advising patients with a history of a heart attack to cut down on cigarette smoking if they have previously been smokers, especially if they have been heavy smokers. Thus, in a general way, there must have been an impression that in some way cigarette smoking is unfavorable with respect to this form of heart disease. However, such advice given to persons who have already had one or more heart attacks may be because of adverse effects anticipated when obvious heart disease is already present. What is of much greater interest is whether or not cigarette smoking is associated with any increase in the tendency to develop heart attacks in persons who have never had one before. Here physicians have, in the past, been less definite, some feeling that cigarette smoking is associated with an excessive risk of future heart attacks, while others were not convinced that this was the case. From what we might call "general experience" there was no clear-cut case either way with regard to cigarette smoking and the risk of future heart attacks.

How does one go about determining whether cigarette smoking is or is not truly associated with an excessive risk of heart disease? Several possible approaches exist, and evidence has now been obtained from careful scientific observation in different ways which clearly does associate cigarette smoking with a predisposition to heart attacks.

First we may consider the evidence derived from the study of persons who have had a heart attack, compared with persons otherwise alike (same age, sex, etc.) who have not yet had any evidence of coronary heart disease. Such a study was made carefully on approximately 100 men who had had a heart attack below the age of forty years compared with healthy men by Drs. Gertler and White. They questioned both groups about their smoking habits. While it was found that both groups smoked cigarettes to some extent, two facts become clearly evident from these studies:

1. The average number of cigarettes habitually smoked per day by the group of heart attack survivors was about 50 per cent higher than the average number of cigarettes smoked per day by the healthy group.

2. There were approximately twice as many nonsmokers among the healthy group as there were in the group of survivors of a heart attack.

These studies certainly show an association of smoking with coronary heart disease, at least within the limits of a study possible by questioning survivors of a heart attack. There are good reasons for not being satisfied with such evidence alone. First of all, there is a chance that the answers given by the heart attack survivors may have, in part, been influenced by their own suspicion that smoking had in some way contributed to their having had a heart attack. Under such circumstances they may have overestimated their average consumption of cigarettes. Furthermore, since this type of study was carried out on survivors of a heart attack, there are missing from the group those persons who had had a heart attack but who had not survived to be able to answer questions concerning their smoking habits. It is conceivable that this may in some way have influenced the conclusion that smoking was more prevalent and in greater amount in persons with a heart attack.

Such evidence, while probably highly indicative, is inconclusive. This brings up the other approach, a far more satisfactory one—a determination of the smoking habits of a large number of persons, preferably tens or hundreds of thousands, at a time when they are healthy, and without any overt evidence of coronary heart disease. Out of such a group there will, with passage of time, grow a number of cases of heart attacks, some surviving, others not. For *these* cases of heart attacks, the smoking history will have been known *in advance* of the heart attack, and hence be uninfluenced by whether or not the person survives the heart attack or by any of his own views concerning the relationship of heart attacks to smoking. In such a study the speed with which one obtains a definitive answer is determined by the number of subjects in the study. The larger the number of healthy people questioned concerning smoking habits, the sooner will there be a sufficient number of heart attacks for the evidence to be analyzed to determine whether or not smokers show a higher heart attack rate (or risk) than do nonsmokers.

Fortunately, this study *has been done* on a very large scale, with highly conclusive results. In a sense the study was not done with this objective as a primary one, but rather because of an interest in a possible relationship of cigarette smoking with cancer of the lung. The American Cancer Society decided to investigate the fate of smokers versus nonsmokers with respect to lung cancer and at the same time with respect to a variety of other disorders, including coronary heart attacks. For these purposes the field workers of the American Cancer Society interviewed over 200,000 persons concerning their smoking habits—that is, whether they smoked, what they smoked (cigarettes, cigars, or pipes) and how much they smoked, on the average. These findings were filed away, and then, of course, during the ensuing months and years a number of heart attacks occurred among the very large number of subjects interviewed.

The early findings of the follow-up period were published by

Dr. E. Hammond and Dr. D. Horn of the Cancer Society in 1954. Their results showed clearly that men in their fifties and sixties who were regular smokers of cigarettes developed approximately 1.5 to 2 times as many heart attacks per thousand men each year as did those men who had never smoked cigarettes. This type of evidence, derived by questioning a large sample of the population *first* and then observing who thereafter develops heart disease, is free of all the criticisms one might have of asking questions of men who have survived one or more heart attacks.

The evidence presented by the Cancer Society hardly leaves any room for doubt or question concerning the fact that heavy cigarette smoking is in some way associated with an excessive heart attack rate. There are some sources which have attempted to belittle these important results of the Cancer Society's study. For example, it is stated that the proof of a higher heart attack rate in cigarette smokers than in nonsmokers does not of *itself* prove that cigarette smoking is one of the *causes* of heart attacks. The reasoning such critics use is that possibly a certain type of individual is prone to have heart attacks and at the same time is the type of person who would take up the smoking of cigarettes. If this were true, his proneness to heart attacks, it is argued, might still exist even if he had never taken up smoking, or had given it up once he had become a smoker. The validity of this *possibility* would not be denied by any sound, scientific thinker. Such a possibility always must be considered in problems such as this. But it would be the most glaring of ostrich-head-in-the-sand techniques to forget the other possibility, which is *at least* equally likely: that cigarette smoking is one of the direct *causes* of increased heart attack rates.

In scientific medical problems such as this, the first step is to test whether or not two things are related, such as cigarette smoking and heart attacks. Then such problems as whether the first item causes the second (here cigarette smoking causing

heart disease) or whether both items are caused by some third
factor (here cigarette smoking and heart disease both being
separate results of the metabolic makeup or personality makeup
of the individual) can be considered by appropriate further
studies. What is extremely important to realize is that the clear-
cut demonstration of an association between cigarette smoking
and coronary heart attacks is a monumental step forward in our
understanding. Even if cigarette smoking does not turn out to
be an actual cause of heart attacks, the information developed
would still be leading us to the identification of some factor in
the makeup of certain individuals that does lead them to an
inordinate susceptibility to heart attacks. Such a lead we can
hardly afford to ignore or overlook.

Knowing now that in some way cigarette smoking *is* associated with an excessive risk of coronary heart attacks, we must
ask ourselves the question whether such an association represents wholly new information concerning heart attacks or
whether it is in some way a reflection of one of the prime
factors previously identified and shown to be associated with
increasing heart attack risk. Let us recall that the two primary
factors identified as increasing heart disease risk by increasing
hardening of the coronary arteries are (1) the amount in the
blood of certain lipoprotein substances and (2) the blood pressure in the arterial system. Now we must determine whether
cigarette smoking is related either to an increase in the average
amount of such lipoproteins in the blood or to an average increase in the person's blood pressure. If cigarette smoking is
associated with changes either in the blood lipoproteins or the
blood pressure, it *does not add* a new primary factor in our
knowledge of heart attacks. If it is *not* associated with a change
either in the lipoproteins or in the blood pressure, cigarette
smoking would represent an additional factor which would require extensive pursuit and elucidation.

These questions—whether cigarette smoking is associated
with any alteration in blood lipoproteins or blood pressure—

can now be answered from *direct experimental measurements* on humans in a large population sample. For this study 2200 consecutive employed persons in apparently good health were asked to fill out a questionnaire concerning their smoking habits at the time when they were undergoing a routine medical examination at their place of employment. These persons had no idea why the questions were being asked or with what other measurements the smoking history was going to be compared. Hence there is essentially no chance that they would have biased their replies in one direction or another. During the medical examination blood pressures were measured in routine fashion and a sample of blood was withdrawn for lipoprotein analysis. When the questionnaire information was used to divide the subjects into categories such as "Never Smoked," "Smoke Cigars and Pipes Only," "Smoke Cigarettes" (this was divided into subcategories depending upon the number of cigarettes smoked per day), the following important facts became clear:

1. Both for men and women, and at every age from twenty to sixty years, cigarette smokers showed a distinctly higher level, on the average, of certain of the blood lipoprotein classes (the S_f 0–12 lipoproteins) than did nonsmokers (those who never smoked). These findings were consistent in each age category studied, and the difference in average lipoprotein level between cigarette smokers and nonsmokers was large enough that chance alone could not have explained the observations even once in a thousand times. It can therefore be regarded as safely *proved* that cigarette smoking is associated with elevation of certain of the blood lipoproteins that are related to coronary arterial hardening and hence to heart attack risk.

2. It was not possible to prove that the average lipoprotein levels were any different in the smokers of pipes or cigars, or both, from the lipoproteins in those persons who had never smoked at all. Why this difference should exist between ciga-

rettes as a source of tobacco smoking and pipes or cigars is not at all clear at present. It may be related to a lesser intake of tobacco in the pipe and cigar smokers than in the cigarette smokers, or even to fillers in the cigarette or to some component of the paper wrapping. It is of interest in this connection that the Cancer Society study showed cigarette smokers to have more heart attacks than cigar or pipe smokers.

3. It could be shown clearly and unequivocally that those persons who had once been smokers of cigarettes *but who had quit* before the time they were studied showed no difference in the amount of lipoproteins in their blood from persons who had never smoked. Therefore if we assume that when they had been smokers of cigarettes they had the elevation in amount of lipoproteins that smokers have, it follows that quitting smoking has resulted in a reduction of their lipoproteins back to the value it would have been had they never smoked. The indication, therefore, is extremely strong that *no matter how* cigarette smoking comes to be associated with elevation of the amount of lipoproteins in the blood, it is possible to overcome this elevation in the lipoproteins of the blood if one stops smoking.

These striking findings show clearly that cigarette smoking in some way is associated with a rise in the amount of certain crucial blood lipoproteins that are themselves associated with increasing the risk of heart disease. Therefore at least part of the effect observed by the Cancer Society study of increased heart attack rates among cigarette smokers can be explained by the fact that cigarette smokers have higher lipoprotein levels, which would lead us to expect a higher heart attack rate. We shall return to the issue of whether or not the effect of smoking on blood lipoproteins accounts for only part of the over-all effect on heart attack risk after the blood pressure factor is considered.

There are some who would immediately deny that smoking cigarettes *causes* the blood lipoprotein elevation. They would admit that cigarette smokers do show the higher lipoprotein values, on the average, but would say that possibly certain types of people have some metabolic or nervous factor that, on the one hand, leads them to smoke cigarettes and, on the other hand, to have high blood levels of these particular lipoproteins. One cannot deny that this interpretation is *possible*, but it is hardly *likely* in the face of all the evidence at hand. First of all, it would require that the amount of "nervous tension" that leads to smoking half a package of cigarettes is only enough to raise the lipoproteins half as much as that which leads to smoking a full package of cigarettes per day. Also, this concept would require that when these persons quit smoking cigarettes their "nervous tension" decreased enough to lower their lipoprotein levels back to those of nonsmokers. All of this is possible, but not likely. What is far more likely, in the author's opinion, is that cigarette smoking somehow affects the control mechanism in the body for the amount of S_f 0–12 lipoproteins in the blood, and the greater the cigarette consumption the more the effect, and the higher the lipoprotein levels. The fact that people who have stopped smoking showed the same lipoprotein levels as those who never smoked suggests strongly that the effect of cigarette smoking on the control mechanism is *reversible*.

Now let us turn our attention to the other major factor in increasing the risk of heart attacks, blood pressure. What is the relationship of cigarette smoking to the blood pressure? Here we have evidence available concerning two different points: (1) the effect on the blood pressure during the act of actually smoking cigarettes and (2) the effect on the blood pressure of habitual smokers (compared with that of nonsmokers) not actually in the act of smoking a cigarette.

In some direct investigations of the blood pressure of some habitual smokers during the act of smoking cigarettes, Dr. Grace Roth found that, on the average, the blood pressure rose 14 points above the base value of 69 points during the actual act of smoking two cigarettes consecutively, a rise of 20 per cent in the blood pressure. However, the pressure had returned to the value it had before smoking the two cigarettes within five minutes. It would appear clear, therefore, that while actually smoking, the average smoker does experience a rise in blood pressure, but the effect wears off rapidly after the act of smoking ceases. This is in good agreement with the measurements of the blood pressures in smokers of cigarettes, compared with that of nonsmokers, made on the individuals at a time they were not actually in the act of smoking a cigarette (usually at least fifteen minutes after smoking the last cigarette). These measurements of the blood pressure were made on the same 2200 consecutive employed persons who were studied for the effect of cigarette smoking on the quantity of the blood lipoproteins. In this study, for every age group of men studied from twenty to sixty years and for women in the age range eighteen to thirty-nine years it was impossible to demonstrate any difference whatever in the average blood pressure (while not in the act of smoking) for heavy cigarette smokers from that of those persons who had never smoked. This finding would confirm the studies of smokers which show that the effect of smoking on the blood pressure is over in approximately five minutes after the cigarette smoking ceases. Since the large-scale study was done while the subjects were not smoking, and at least fifteen minutes after the last cigarette, it is not surprising that no effect was found of cigarette smoking on blood pressure.

Thus, in summary we can say that (1) while actually smoking cigarettes the blood pressure is raised on the average, and (2) during the period when the person is not actually smoking, there is no effect of habitual smoking on the blood pressure.

How do we handle this information with respect to the smoking–blood pressure relationships to assess its role in the development of heart attacks? We know that if the blood pressure is elevated, the risk of future heart attacks is clearly higher than if the blood pressure is not elevated—this has been con-clusively proved (see Chapter 7). But cigarette smoking ele-vates blood pressure only while the cigarette is smoked and for a short time thereafter (approximately five minutes). It would be expected that the elevation of the pressure for part of each day would have approximately a proportionate effect upon the heart attack risk. Thus, for example, if we consider a man who smokes two packages of cigarettes per day (forty cigarettes), he will have the smoking effect on blood pressure for ten minutes for each cigarette, on the average, or a total of 400 minutes per day, which is approximately seven hours out of each twenty-four-hour day. If the average elevation of blood pressure is 14 points for smoking cigarettes, then we could say such a man has $\frac{7}{24}$ of 14, spread over the twenty-four hours, or an equivalent of 4 points of average increase in blood pres-sure. From risk calculations relating blood pressure to heart attacks, a 4-point elevation in blood pressure corresponds to multiplying the heart attack rate by 1.4 (a 40 per cent in-crease), on the average.

But we must also consider the effect of cigarette smoking in raising the blood lipoproteins and Atherogenic Index, which separately increases the risk of future heart attacks. Risk calcu-lations show that this effect of cigarette smoking on lipo-proteins would itself multiply the heart attack rate by 1.5, on the average, for smokers of forty cigarettes per day (a 50 per cent increase). The over-all effect of smoking forty cigarettes per day on heart attack rate is obtained, to a good first approxi-mation, by multiplying the blood pressure effect by the Athero-genic Index effect. Therefore, smokers of forty cigarettes per day (two packs) would be expected to show 2.1 times as many heart attacks as nonsmokers (obtained by multiplying 1.5 by 1.4). The Cancer Society statistics show directly that regular smokers of forty cigarettes per day have approximately 2.2 times as many heart attacks as do nonsmokers. The agreement between the predicted value of 2.1 and the observed value of

2.2 for excessive heart attacks among heavy smokers is astoundingly close. Considering the experimental errors in both measurements, it is entirely possible that the true agreement is perfect, which would mean that the relationship of cigarette smoking to excessive heart attack rate is wholly explained by the higher blood lipoproteins and higher blood pressure in the cigarette smokers. Certainly, if the effect is not wholly explained in this way, the greatest part of the effect is so explained.

CHAPTER 12

Emotional Stress, Occupation, Physical Activity, and Heart Attacks

We are said to live in an age of society's history where the stresses upon man are greater than they ever were before. Undoubtedly, people of many generations have been equally certain that the stresses of "modern living" of their generation were greater than they ever had been before or ever would be again. Whether we, in the twentieth century, are truly subjected to emotional tension or stress by our pace of living that exceeds anything ever before known is very difficult to assess. Primarily it is difficult to assess because there exists no good or universally acceptable way even to approximate the degree of emotional stress or tension a person is under over an average hour, day, week, month, year, or lifetime. What one person might consider a stressful situation another might thrive on and consider relaxation. Certainly if any authorities on the subject have told us how to measure emotional tension and stress in each person, they have hidden the directions for such measurements extremely well. As a result, the entire field of evaluating the possible effects of life stresses and emotional tension on health or disease is a very muddy field, itself studded with opinions, emotions and other substitutions for valid scientific evaluation. Often an opinion is offered that a par-

137

ticular disease event in a person was caused by a stressful situation. When that opinion is questioned because of inadequacy of the evidence, the reaction is that the person questioning the opinion "cannot tolerate this explanation" because he himself is subjected to this same type of stress but does not want to face it. With this type of answer to a question concerning the method of establishing causes of disease, the situation is hopeless for a really valid scientific or statistical approach, since the approach itself is not admitted. Thus circular reasoning, without supporting evidence, can go on ad infinitum, never provable, but always present to muddy any real effort to arrive at the truth that may underlie such problems.

The problem of occurrence of coronary heart attacks is very much in the current limelight of this area of concern over emotional tension, life stress, and the pace of "modern living." First, it seems quite clear from the available statistics that heart attacks have increased in frequency in the United States and certain other Western countries, such as Great Britain, during the past half-century. This seems to be true, even after correcting for such factors as better diagnostic methods in heart disease and for the fact that more people are now living to the age range where heart attacks occur frequently. In other words, there does appear to have occurred a real increase in the heart attack rate, especially in men, over this span of years. It is only natural that many private theories will emerge concerning the cause of this increase.

Further, it is not unexpected, in an age of rapid scientific and technological development, that the "increased pace of living" should be blamed for the increase in heart attacks, especially since there is very little that is not being laid these days at the door of "the stress of modern life." Thus, executives of industry, hearing of or knowing of a fellow-executive of their own or another corporation having had a heart attack at forty-five years of age, soon begin to feel certain that premature heart attacks are the fate of *all* executives and of hardly anyone else. This is understandable, since the executive travels in a world of other executives and would hardly be expected to know of premature heart attacks in laborers, clerks, or farmers. Similarly, the busy physician sees other physicians having heart attacks, and because he is overburdened with a heavy practice begins to feel sure that the "strain" of the practice and the responsibility which goes with it must be the basis for "so many" heart attacks among physicians. A large part of the reason why so many groups come to feel that heart attacks are so frequent among their colleagues is that (1) they know their colleagues, and (2) heart attacks do represent a very common disease—indeed, the leading cause of death of men above thirty-five years of age.

Tremendous emotional pressure lies behind this desire to blame on the stress and strain of modern life the occurrence of heart attacks. In some quarters it is even dangerous to disagree with this preconceived notion. At a recent medical meeting attended by the author, one speaker, with much fervor, asked the audience of doctors for a show of hands as to how many thought the stress of modern living was the basis for heart attacks. The enthusiastic show of many hands pleased the speaker. One gained the impression that he thought this *proved* the point. Unfortunately, however, *nature* does not behave in a manner to conform to a voting majority of those who attend a medical meeting, and in matters such as science a large voting majority can be wrong if emotions rather than fact may be the basis for the position taken.

But, as with other aspects of the heart attack problem, one cannot afford to overlook possibilities even where emotion rather than factual experience may be the primary basis for the evidence. The old adage "Where there is smoke, there is fire" needs to be heeded, until enough real evidence can be gathered to decide the issue one way or another. Let us, therefore, look at the actual evidence.

One inroad on this problem can be made through some direct studies of occupational categories in relation to heart attack rate. If certain occupations are more stressful to an individual than others, and *if* we assume that such stress carries over into the rest of the daily life of the individual concerned, it should be possible to show that certain occupational categories have higher heart attack rates than others. Even if occupations do show a difference, it would remain to be demonstrated that the occupational *stress* was the factor, or even one factor, involved in the difference. Nevertheless, the first step is to determine whether or not a difference exists. Dr. J. N. Morris, in England, has interested himself in this problem and has made some extremely interesting and pertinent observations. He pointed out, as have many others, that coronary heart attacks are far more common in "highly civilized," prosperous Western populations than among more primitive peoples such as rural Guatemalans, Bantus in South Africa, Okinawans, Ugandan natives, and others. He recognized the factor that diets are grossly different for the inhabitants of prosperous Western countries from those for the primitive peoples (see Chapter 10), but raised the question as to whether multiple other factors in the way of life for primitive peoples might not be more important than their limited diets.

In some direct observations Morris showed, within London, England (so that gross geographic differences do not operate), that the drivers of buses showed a higher attack rate than did the conductors of the same buses, even though they were in comparable age brackets. He found, furthermore, that heart attacks were of a more serious type in the bus drivers than in the conductors. Realizing that this might be a rather special group of persons, Morris extended his investigations to include a variety of other occupations, contrasting heart attack rates in clerks and postmen, farmers and laborers in the city, general practitioners and physicians who were specialists. The observations of Morris for a variety of occupational groups, in addition to his studies of the London transport workers, showed the following results, with the occupations ranked according to heart attack death rate.

Heart attack death rate versus occupational category (all men in the 45–64 year age group)

Occupational category	Heart attack deaths per million people per year
Hairdressers, etc.	880
Makers of textile goods	770
Typists and other clerks (non-Civil Service)	730
Fitters mechanics, toolmakers, etc.	560
Messenger and porters, etc.	500
Railway engine drivers	480
Postmen and sorters	460
Boot and shoe makers, repairers	450
Smiths and skilled forge makers	420
Metal machinists	380
Coal hewers and getters	290
Water transport dock laborers	270
Coal mine workers below ground, except hewers and getters	230
Other workers in building, etc.	170
Agricultural gardeners, laborers, etc.	150

The differences listed here in heart attack rate for the various occupational categories in England are very large. Such differences would be extremely unlikely to arise through measurement errors, sampling errors, or incorrect classification of occupational groups. We can, with a very high degree of assurance, consider that these differences in heart attack rate are real. At this point, though, facts cease to help us and interpretation enters the picture. It becomes vital to understand the possible basis for the observed differences in heart attack rates in the various occupational categories. Since so many factors may differentiate both people and activities in various occupational groups, it is evident that *interpretation* of the significance of the various possible factors is inevitable, and that such interpretation can to a large extent be shaded by personal opinion on the part of the interpreter.

In his considerations of the higher heart attack rate among

the London bus drivers than among the conductors, Morris has pointed out that the drivers, seated in their occupational activity for some eight hours of every working day, have far less physical activity at work than do the bus conductors. The London buses are double-deckers and the conductors make many trips per day up and down the stairs of these buses. When he reviewed the extent of physical activity at work for the many other occupational categories studied, Morris further noted that in general the occupations associated with a high degree of physical activity at work showed a lower heart attack rate than did the occupations associated with a modest or low degree of physical activity at work. The immediate and apparently obvious conclusion that would be drawn from these observations is that occupations requiring physical exertion seem protective against heart attacks in contrast to those requiring less physical exertion. Indeed, on other grounds, there are many who voice the opinion that physical exercise is a major protective influence against the occurrence of heart attacks, a point by no means completely documented as yet. Such comments concerning a possible effect of physical exertion in protection against heart attacks may come as a surprise to some. There exists a common impression that heart attacks may be *precipitated* by unusual physical exertion, such as in persons during or after shoveling snow following a heavy snowstorm. *Unusual* physical exertion in one who is ordinarily sedentary may well be an unfavorable factor, but even in such a case it is certain that extensive hardening of the coronary arteries would already be present. Such excessive physical exertion is by no means a usual precipitating factor in occurrence of heart attacks, for a large proportion of the attacks awaken people out of their sleep after an apparently usual day of their life.

But the physical-exertion explanation of these observations is hardly the only one that has been advanced, or could be advanced. Thus, for the case of the bus drivers versus the bus conductors, Morris himself has raised the question whether other totally different explanations may not be more reasonable than that of physical exertion. The drivers, he has pointed out, are constantly in the midst of congested London traffic and might be subjected to a great deal of mental and emotional stress during each working day, a stress that may be regarded as less prevalent for the bus conductors. This difference in mental or emotional stress, he has pointed out, deserves consideration as an explanation for the difference in heart attack rates between drivers and conductors. Although the question of just how stressful traffic is to a bus driver has never been quantitated, it does seem *intuitively* possible that such stress is greater than it is for a conductor. This possible explanation for the observations cannot be ruled out summarily. On the other hand, he indicated that the difference in heart attack rates between clerks and postmen is not so readily blamed on "obvious" stressful situations in their daily work life, nor can obvious stress be the explanation for all the other occupational differences.

One of the real dilemmas of a problem such as this arises out of the difficulty of measuring stress in a clerk and in a postman. No doubt *with* the knowledge that clerks have a higher incidence of heart attacks than do postmen, those who lean toward the concept that "emotional, mental, or life stress" is important in development of heart attacks could readily develop for us a beautiful case to demonstrate how stressful the life of a clerk is, compared with that of a postman. The only difficulty with this is that we can be reasonably certain that if it had turned out that the postmen had higher heart attack rates than the clerks, these same authorities could have made out an equally impressive case for the greater stresses of living on the postmen than on the clerks. Such "fitting the facts" after one knows *how* the facts need to be fitted will plague us forever on this issue as long as the evaluation of emotional and life stress is so completely subjective, rather than quantitative and objective. This in no way denies the possible importance of the emotional stress of living, but simply points up the fact that there is room for a large contribution to medical science in the form of at least a beginning of an approach to real *measurement* in this particular field.

Even considerations of emotional stress and physical exertion hardly end the significant possibilities for the explanation of the differing heart attack rates observed among the different occupational groups. There is the all-important question of *what type of person* chooses to go into a particular occupation. It might not be unexpected that the type of person who becomes a clerk (together with his eating pattern, smoking habits, and hereditary chemical makeup) may be very different from the type of person who becomes a postman, a bus conductor, or a laborer.

Some one of these factors (type of person, stress, or physical activity) or one not yet mentioned may well be the basis for the difference in heart attack rates observed among the various occupational groups. Whichever one should turn out to be correct, there would immediately arise the question as to the mechanism by which it operates. We know that two solidly established factors exist in determining heart attack risk, the amount in the blood of certain lipoproteins and the level of the blood pressure. Does physical activity or emotional stress or some such factor operate to alter the average amount of lipoproteins in the blood or to alter the average level of the blood pressure in the person? *If it does*, we should not be at all surprised to find a different heart attack rate in groups differing widely in either emotional stress or physical activity.

It has been long known to physiology and to medicine that emotional stress and physical activities can have profound effects upon the chemical and nervous systems of the body. The existence of such chemical and nervous effects means it would not be difficult to believe that the regulation either of the level of the amount of blood lipoproteins or of the blood pressure would thereby be affected. This type of possibility can be looked at directly for various occupational groups, since both the lipoprotein values and the blood pressures are available for large numbers of men in a variety of occupational categories. Such values are tabulated below, according to occupational categories, from the large-scale periodic medical examinations in one particular industrial activity where a wide variety of occupations was represented. The advantage of studying a single industrial activity is that all the individuals concerned have to a large extent a common environment at work, at least with respect to certain factors such as geographic location, weather, and a host of others. The various occupational categories are listed below in the order of those showing the highest average Atherogenic Index values (which is the combined measure of the blood lipoproteins) through successive categories of lower Atherogenic Index values. In some of the occupational categories there were relatively small numbers of persons available for examination, so that the average Atherogenic Index value is not so well fixed as for occupational categories with large numbers of persons examined. Therefore the number of cases examined will be tabulated, together with comments concerning which differences in Atherogenic Index between groups are sufficiently large that sampling alone is not likely to account for the observed differences. Also, since the average age of each occupational category was not identical, all the values have been appropriately adjusted to the value for the age of thirty-five years. Only men are considered in this tabulation.

In reviewing these findings it is necessary to remember that small differences in average Atherogenic Index values between any two occupational categories may be chance occurrences, especially if the number of cases studied in one or another occupational category is small. But some of the differences noted in the above tabulation are not small; they are startling. This feature can be underlined by noting that a group of in-

Atherogenic Index (lipoprotein) values in various occupational categories (listed from highest values to lowest)

Occupational category	Number of men studied	Average Atherogenic Index value (in units)
Operators of computers or duplicating machines	21	80.6
Truck and bus drivers	23	79.6
Tool and die makers (machinists)	62	77.1
Firemen	17	75.0
Painters	13	75.0
Journeyman machinists	70	74.5
Laboratory technicians	40	73.9
Mathematicians	54	72.7
Carpenters	20	71.6
Mechanical technicians	80	70.8
Machinists and machinists' helpers	57	70.4
Welders	14	70.4
Junior and assistant executives	58	70.0
Engineers	244	69.3
Clerks	20	69.0
Draftsmen	99	68.7
Electricians	41	68.5
Electronic technicians	147	68.3
Steamfitters and boiler operators	21	68.0
Chemists	70	67.7
Physicists	217	67.5
Police officers	80	65.8
Operators of accelerator machines	62	64.7
Storehouse workers	31	62.2
Laborers	36	61.4
Custodians	42	57.0
Sheet metal workers	21	54.3

dividuals with an average Atherogenic Index value of 75 units will be expected, all other things being equal, to show about two times as many heart attacks per one thousand men per year as a group with an average Atherogenic Index of 55 units.

Such differences among the occupational categories listed above are quite definitely real. For example, a comparison of the tool and die maker machinists, a group which shows high Atherogenic Index values, with the laborers or the custodians, both of which groups show low Atherogenic Index values, indicates that there is less than one chance in a thousand that the difference between the machinists and either of the two low groups could be the result of the sampling alone. Therefore we are very much assured that the differences are real.

Why some of the phenomenal differences in Atherogenic Index exist between certain of these occupational categories is quite another matter, not so readily resolved as the discovery of the differences themselves. Numerous possible explanations come to mind, some of which may be subjected to direct test and others of which would be difficult to test objectively with presently available methods. An investigator such as Dr. Morris could look at this tabulation of values and point out that two groups who do a great deal of heavy *physical* work in their occupation, laborers and custodians, are near the bottom of the list of Atherogenic Index values. This would be consistent with his finding that heavy physical labor is characteristic of those occupations in which the heart attack rate is relatively low.

On the other hand, this aspect of the story certainly appears to have some inconsistencies in it. For example, tool and die maker machinists would appear to have more physical activity in their work than theoretical physicists, who work largely at a desk with pencil and paper. Out of the group of 217 physicists there were forty-five clearly designated as theoretical physicists, and their average Atherogenic Index was calculated to be 65.1 units. This value of 65.1 is *lower* than the 77.1 value for the tool and die maker machinists. If physical activity of occupation were *the* crucial issue, we would have expected a reversal of these averages. The criticism might be raised that a comparison of machinists and physicists with respect to physical activity in work is unfair because other factors may differentiate these two groups. A more appropriate comparison can be made within the group of physicists. It is extremely likely that there is more physical activity at work for experimental physicists than for theoretical physicists. If physical activity is *the* issue, the theoretical physicists would be expected to show a *higher* average Atherogenic Index than the other physicists. By actual test the forty-five theoretical physicists showed an average

Atherogenic Index value of 65.1 units, whereas the remaining 172 physicists showed an average Atherogenic Index value of 68.3 units. Thus, if anything, the theoretical physicists showed slightly lower values than the others, although the physical-activity concept would have led us to expect them to show higher values.

In summary, it can be said that while physical activity of occupation may *in part* account for the different Atherogenic Index values among occupational categories, other factors must be operative which at times can overshadow this one.

Investigators who lean toward the concept that emotional, mental, or life stress explains the risk of heart attacks would undoubtedly be able to explain the differing Atherogenic Index averages among the occupational categories in terms of the stresses of the occupations. They might point out that tool and die maker machinists, who are highly skilled workers with exacting demands in their work and with a high order of responsibility, would be expected to show higher average Atherogenic Index values than would heavy laborers or custodians with lesser demands of an exacting or responsible type. This seems quite straightforward, once one knows that the tool and die makers do show higher Atherogenic Index values than do the laborers and custodians. It would be much more convincing if one could rate such features as frustration, exacting demands of the work, ambition, mental stress, and responsibility on a measuring scale and *then* look at the rated categories to see if the Atherogenic Index values fit.

Some preliminary tests of the concept of the effect of responsibility, demands, and stress have been made in the occupational categories under study, and these certainly lend no support to this theory. Taking several occupational categories together, individuals have been selected out who are listed as supervisors, foremen, or coordinators, all of which are special-responsibility positions. The average Atherogenic Index value for a group of sixty-two such individuals was 68.6 units while for the occupational categories out of which they were selected the average was 70.0 units. Thus, rather than showing higher Atherogenic Index values, the supervisory personnel had a value slightly though not significantly lower than the nonsupervisory personnel in the same occupational categories. As another test of the effect of responsibility of position, the entire group of engineers was divided into subgroups based upon their professional ratings. Higher professional ratings are accompanied by increased responsibility, demands, and a higher income. After correcting for the effect of age in the various categories so that the values are all corrected to thirty-five years of age, no significant difference was found to exist in the average Atherogenic Index values for the engineers with the lowest professional ratings, for those with intermediate ratings, or for those with the highest ratings. If such factors as responsibility, demands, and frustration are important here, probably we need some better techniques for their evaluation before any definitive answers can be given concerning the possible effects of these stresses on Atherogenic Index values.

There do exist certain other objective possibilities that may explain the Atherogenic Index differences among occupational categories. Among these are factors that have clearly been identified in previous chapters as being definitely important in determining the level of the Atherogenic Index. They are the following:

1. The dietary habits of individuals, especially with respect to the daily intake of carbohydrate or of animal and saturated vegetable fats.
2. The incidence of overweight, since it is clear that overweight is, on the average, associated with elevation of the Atherogenic Index.
3. The cigarette smoking habit, since it has been clearly shown that the average heavy cigarette smoker has higher lipoprotein levels and a higher Atherogenic Index value than the nonsmoker.

It is entirely possible that further studies of the various occupational categories may show significant differences in diet, weight, or smoking habits and that these differences may account in part or completely for the observed differences in Atherogenic Index. In any event, these three factors can be tested objectively and without emotional or personal bias on the part of the investigator seeking an answer.

We may now turn our attention to the other major factor in determination of the risk of coronary heart attacks. Can occupation have an effect of consequence on the blood pressure? The same type of analysis of blood pressures for the various occupational categories has been made as that for the Atherogenic Index value. In the table below the average blood pressure values for each of the occupational categories studied are presented, listed from the highest values to the lowest.

Blood pressure values in various occupational categories (listed from highest values to lowest)

Occupational category	Number of men studied	Average blood pressure
Painters	13	75.4
Firemen	17	73.6
Clerks	20	73.5
Machinists and machinists' helpers	57	73.3
Carpenters	20	72.9
Storehouse workers	31	71.8
Draftsmen	99	71.5
Journeyman machinists	70	71.4
Laboratory technicians	40	71.3
Truck and bus drivers	23	71.2
Tool and die makers (machinists)	62	70.8
Chemists	70	70.7
Mathematicians	54	70.7
Junior and assistant executives	58	70.6
Operators of computers or duplicating machines	21	70.6
Electronic technicians	147	70.5
Physicists	217	70.4
Steamfitters and boiler operators	21	70.2
Operators of accelerator machines	62	70.2
Police officers	80	70.1
Mechanical technicians	80	70.0
Engineers	244	69.9
Custodians	42	69.5
Electricians	41	69.5
Laborers	36	69.2
Sheet metal workers	21	67.1
Welders	14	66.0

Upon inspection of this table one is struck immediately by the very small range exhibited by the average blood pressures from the occupational categories with the highest recorded averages to those with the lowest recorded averages. Furthermore, at the two ends of the table where the high or low values occur, we note that there are only small numbers of cases. It would not be surprising that by chance sampling of a small group one could run into this amount of difference from the highest group to the lowest. Careful statistical analysis of these averages shows:

1. Even the highest average value, 75.4, for painters cannot be proved to be significantly different from the lowest recorded average values, 66.0, for welders. Chance sampling could account for this difference.
2. No pair of occupational groups can be proved to have different average blood pressures.
3. No occupational category can be proved from this evidence to have an average blood pressure different from the group as a whole.

There is, therefore, a striking absence of any effect of occupational category upon the blood pressure. This will surely prove disappointing to many who believe, without good evidence, that occupational stress must surely affect the blood pressure. It would certainly appear that among these twenty-seven widely different occupational categories any difference in occupational stress sufficient to affect blood pressure would have revealed itself. The possibility remains, of course, that emotional or mental stresses in certain occupations as well as in other facets of life might *temporarily* raise the blood pressure and thus have a proportionate effect on heart attack risk, but certainly occupation is, from this evidence, not associated with any measurable sustained effects on the blood pressure.

In summary, the evidence appears good that certain occupations are associated with excessive heart attack risk. Further, certain occupations show appreciable differences in Atherogenic Index values, which would lead to an expectation of differing heart attack risks. While physical activity of occupation may be one reason for such differences, it does not appear to be an adequate explanation for all the differences. The explanation of differing heart attack risks and Atherogenic Index values for the various occupations in terms of job stress, frustrations, responsibility, or similar features cannot be supported from any of the evidence developed. If emotional or life stress is a factor in heart attack risks, it will probably require waiting for some reasonable way to measure these stresses to prove any real effect.

CHAPTER 13

Relationship of Diabetes to Heart Attacks

Diabetes mellitus, commonly referred to simply as "diabetes" or "sugar diabetes," has widely been considered to be associated with premature hardening of the arteries, coronary and other, and with an excessive risk of heart attacks. Many statements have been made that the discovery of insulin as a specific treatment for diabetes has almost wholly eliminated the reason for anyone ever dying of diabetes itself, but that such complications as hardening of the coronary arteries and premature heart attacks still exist in the diabetic patient in spite of the widespread use of insulin. It would, of course, be expected that diabetic persons, like other persons in the population at large, should develop coronary artery narrowing and should have some heart attacks. It would not be expected that the discovery of insulin should have removed from the diabetic *all* risk of the single most common disease that kills adult Americans. The real issue is whether diabetics today show a higher incidence of heart attacks than do nondiabetics of the same sex and age in the population.

That diabetics once had more hardening of the arteries and more frequent heart attacks, during the preinsulin era, seems to be reasonably well substantiated from a variety of sources of evidence. That diabetics today have more hardening of the

arteries and more frequent heart attacks is a much more difficult point to establish. There is great difficulty in establishing
the true status of diabetics today with respect to heart attacks.
First of all, there is the question of recognized and treated
diabetes versus unrecognized and untreated diabetes. This disease is estimated to exist in something over a million persons
in the United States who do not even know they are diabetics,
in spite of the ease with which the disease can be discovered
through very simple urine and blood tests. For these unrecognized and untreated diabetics any predisposition to hardening
of the arteries that characterizes diabetes would still exist, for
they would not even have had an opportunity to benefit from
any effect that treatment may have in reduction of the rate of
hardening of the arteries and the risk of heart attacks. Even
if they finally are discovered and treated for their diabetes, they
may have spent years and even decades untreated, therefore
developing coronary artery hardening at the rate for untreated
diabetes. If, therefore, untreated diabetes does predispose to
heart attacks, it will not be surprising to see its effects even
during this insulin era. To be sure, it is not likely that a very
severe diabetic will go on for many years without discovery
and treatment simply because the severity of his illness would
force recognition, but many of the moderate cases can and do
escape notice.

Further difficulties cloud the true picture of the risk of coronary heart disease in diabetics today. It is commonly forgotten
that insulin only came into use approximately thirty years ago,
and its acceptance and wide medical use were not instantaneous.
Therefore, during the past ten years diabetic patients who are
considered medically may have spent an appreciable part of
their life effectively in the preinsulin period. If, during that
part of their life, hardening of the arteries was proceeding at
an accelerated rate, it can be anticipated that some of the
results would be affecting the heart disease status of sixty- and
seventy-year-old diabetics of the past ten years, in spite of

widespread current usage of insulin. Therefore, evidence purporting to show that modern-day treatment of diabetes with insulin has not helped curb hardening of the arteries or has not helped reduce the risk of heart disease is extremely suspect, especially when based on evidence concerning sixty- or seventy-year-old diabetics over the past ten-year period. This is not just a hypothetical concern, since many of the published medical reports concerning hardening of the arteries and heart disease in diabetics have been based upon studies of seventy- and eighty-year-old diabetics, which is even worse.

Another common fallacy noted in statements concerning the incidence of heart attacks in diabetics centers around failure to recognize the effect of age itself. Diabetes of the usual form is relatively more common in the middle and later years than in the early years of life, although it may occur even in children. As a result the average diabetic individual is older than the average person in the population at large. Since heart attacks increase in frequency with increasing age, this fact alone would lead to a higher heart attack rate in the diabetic population than in the nondiabetic population. It is surprising how frequently this age factor is overlooked in writings on this subject.

With respect to the fully treated diabetic there is still major controversy among eminent specialists in this field as to whether the fully treated diabetic does or does not show any increase in risk of heart attacks. In those clinics where it is believed that careful management of the diabetics removes the excessive risk of heart disease ascribed to diabetes, the opinion is frequently voiced that the reason for any excess frequency of heart attacks in diabetics is the inadequate degree of treatment of the diabetes itself. In those clinics where it is believed that treated diabetics still carry an excessive risk of heart attacks, the occurrence of heart attacks in diabetics is regarded simply as corroborative evidence supporting their point of view.

For the diabetic person all this is very far from an academic argument. He would like very much to know whether it is true that diabetes per se, treated or untreated, predestines him to an excessive risk of coronary heart attacks. An intelligent answer to his question would start with consideration of the problem of how diabetes might in any way have come to be considered to be a disease predisposing to hardening of the arteries and to heart attacks. Is it some new and unexplained feature of diabetes itself that predisposes to heart disease or may diabetes operate, as we have seen other states operate, through an effect of elevation of the blood lipoproteins (and hence the Atherogenic Index) or the blood pressure, or both? These latter two factors we know to be the major independent factors that truly are associated with increasing the rate of hardening of the arteries and the risk of heart attacks. If diabetes should operate only through the lipoprotein elevation or the blood pressure elevation or both, then an enormous load could be taken off the mind of the members of our diabetic population. No longer would the *word* diabetes carry the threat to life of a possible premature heart attack. Replacing this would be the easy task of measurement of the blood lipoproteins and blood pressure. If these two measurements were favorably low, the diabetic would then have no reason to feel that he has any excessive risk of heart disease. Indeed, his risk might be considerably lower than that for the average person of the same age in the population at large. Many diabetic persons do show low lipoprotein levels in the blood and normal or low blood pressures. For them the issue of whether the diabetes *itself* is an additional hazard with respect to heart disease risk is paramount.

First, is diabetes in any way associated with elevation of the lipoproteins or the Atherogenic Index? Here we must ask "Diabetes *in what phase?*" before attempting to answer. Diabetes is a state which can vary in severity in a single person, for a variety of reasons. When the severity of the diabetes increases, as it may, for example, during infection, the diabetes is said to be in a state of decontrol. If this decontrol is not caught early and treated adequately, it is a self-perpetuating and self-accelerating process. The person involved can finally pass into a state of coma.

Many diabetic patients have been studied carefully during periods of varying degrees of decontrol of their disease. Startling and massive changes in the blood lipoproteins occur during the decontrol phase of diabetes. Sometimes diabetics go into this phase of decontrol and finally are brought into a hospital in coma simply because it was not previously known that they were diabetics or because it was not realized that they were slipping more and more into this decontrol phase. All of this can happen in a period of a few days in some cases. When diabetics in this severe decontrol phase with coma are studied, it is found that many of them (the majority, in fact) have extremely high Atherogenic Index values. In one such patient the Atherogenic Index value reached over 800 units, compared with an average value of approximately 75 units in adult males of the population at large. Atherogenic Index values of 200 or 300 are commonly encountered in diabetic patients during severe decontrol or during coma. It should be clear that with such Atherogenic Index values the rate of development of hardening of the coronary arteries would be increased tremendously. There exists some special evidence to indicate that this should be expected.

Some of the diabetics in the severe decontrol phase develop a crop of yellow lumps in their skin, known as *xanthomas* (*xanth*, yellow; *oma*, lump). When examined microscopically, these yellow lumps are noted to represent a fatty deposition in the skin that is almost identical with the fatty deposition that is so prominent a feature of the hardening of arteries such as the coronary arteries. It is quite clear that the reason these yellow lumps form in the skin of diabetics during the severe decontrol phase is that the blood lipoproteins and Atherogenic Index are so enormously elevated at such times. It would be anticipated that the coronary arteries would suffer excessive fatty deposition also as a result of this enormous Atherogenic Index elevation.

Fortunately, this entire process of massive elevation in lipoprotein and Atherogenic Index values is reversible when the diabetes is once again brought under control by medical measures. Repeatedly it has been found that when a comatose diabetic is treated with standard medical methods the markedly elevated Atherogenic Index begins almost immediately to decline sharply. With each passing day the Atherogenic Index falls further, until in a matter of a couple of weeks it may have returned to a value not different from the average values seen in nondiabetics. Even a value such as the Atherogenic Index that reached 800 units during severe decontrol was found to decline to below 100 as the diabetes responded to medical treatment. In those cases in which the yellow lumps, or xanthomas, had formed while the Atherogenic Index was elevated, it was noted that no further xanthomas developed when the Atherogenic Index declined and, further, the xanthomas that were present began to shrink in size and finally disappeared.

In the era before insulin was introduced into medical practice such episodes of severe diabetic decontrol were extremely common and were difficult to treat medically. Many diabetics died during such episodes of severe decontrol because no medical measures were effective. With the availability of insulin this type of diabetic death has become relatively rare, and many authorities feel such deaths should almost never occur now.

In the preinsulin era many diabetics were constantly in varying stages of decontrol. During such decontrol we can be sure they were carrying extremely high Atherogenic Index values in their blood. Therefore they undoubtedly were developing hardening of the coronary arteries at a rapid rate. There is little wonder that heart attacks should have been quite prevalent in the diabetic person of the preinsulin era. Indeed, it would be much more surprising if heart attacks had not been excessive in diabetic persons during the preinsulin era, but this era is fortunately now in the past. Diabetics by and large can be kept out of severely decontrolled phases, especially if they are co-operative in the management of their disease. An obvious and sufficient reason for an excessive heart attack risk—the massive lipoprotein–Atherogenic Index elevation—now is vanishing. Studies of large numbers of diabetics who attend diabetic clinics have been made in recent years and it has been found that their Atherogenic Index values are only slightly elevated, on the average, above those in the population at large. Many diabetics have even lower Atherogenic Index values during good diabetic control than do many nondiabetics of the same age and sex.

So far as the lipoprotein–Atherogenic Index factor is concerned, diabetics need not in general be predisposed to heart attacks in this era. What about other factors? It is common knowledge in medicine that the usual form of diabetes which is seen occurs in middle age in persons who are appreciably overweight. A frequent accompaniment of the overweight and the diabetes in such persons is an elevation of the blood pressure.

Such diabetics have two factors operative that would tend to increase their risk of future coronary heart attacks. First, they are overweight and hence will show, on the average, an elevation of the Atherogenic Index which is associated with the overweight state in general. This elevation in Atherogenic Index will not be anywhere near so great as that which characterizes the state of severe diabetic decontrol.

Second, the elevation in blood pressure is a known factor which increases the rate of coronary arterial narrowing and the risks of future heart attacks. For the very common type of diabetes encountered nowadays there are good and sufficient reasons in the overweight–Atherogenic Index–Blood Pressure Elevation triad for any excessive heart disease risk they may have. Many of these overweight middle-aged diabetics find that their diabetes is brought under control *without* insulin, their elevated blood pressures fall, and the Atherogenic Index declines if they reduce their food intake and thus correct their overweight.

In all of this discussion no mention has been made of something about diabetes *itself* which predisposes to an excessive heart disease risk. The reason for this is that there exists no valid scientific medical evidence that any such feature of diabetes per se exists. The ways in which Atherogenic Index and blood pressure elevation can alter the outlook of a diabetic have been described. These phenomena are well documented. But any statement that there exists some feature of diabetes itself which creates an excessive risk of heart attacks, other than through the blood lipoproteins and blood pressure, is simply speculation with no valid evidence behind it. Recently published evidence on the occurrence of heart attacks in diabetics strongly supports the view that the blood lipoprotein elevation when present is the prime factor in any excessive risk of heart attacks in diabetics. In that study blood lipoproteins were measured in over 500 diabetic patients in a clinic. During the ensuing two to five years a certain number of these diabetic patients suffered heart attacks. It was found that those diabetics who did develop heart attacks had originally had blood lipoprotein elevations over those who did not develop heart attacks. These elevations were comparable in extent to the blood lipoprotein elevation observed in persons of the population at large who develop heart attacks. If there had been some feature of diabetes itself which predisposes to heart attacks, with some diabetics having more of this feature than others, it would have been expected that for a diabetic to develop a heart attack a *lesser* elevation of the blood lipoproteins would have been observed than is the case for nondiabetic persons. Since such was *not* observed, this study of diabetics lends no support to the concept that the diabetes per se predisposes the person to an excessive risk of heart attacks.

In summary, it can be stated that diabetes derives its association with any excessive heart attack risk either from the blood lipoprotein–Atherogenic Index elevation or the blood pressure elevation frequently noted in overweight diabetics. The Atherogenic Index elevation was undoubtedly appreciable during the era before insulin was introduced into medicine, because severe diabetic decontrol was then frequent. Now that such decontrol is relatively rare, the marked elevations in Atherogenic Index are infrequent and it would be expected that heart attack frequency, when properly measured, will no longer be as high as in the diabetics of the preinsulin era. No good evidence exists that diabetes itself, associated with moderate lipoprotein values and blood pressures, predisposes to any excessive heart attack risk. Therefore it is erroneous to assign to a diabetic person an excessive risk of heart attack simply because he is a diabetic. The diabetic, like any other person, can know by blood lipoprotein analysis and blood pressure measurement whether he carries any excessive risk of heart disease. Great numbers of diabetics do not have any excessive risk of heart attacks.

CHAPTER 14

A Program for the Prevention of Heart Attacks

In all the foregoing chapters the various types of information that we *do have* concerning heart attacks have been presented and analyzed for the reader. It should be quite evident that heart attacks no longer represent the mystery that they have been purported to represent in so many pronouncements by both lay and medical persons. A tremendous amount of information *is* available concerning heart attacks. Furthermore, such information has been woven together into a consistent picture with valid, quantitative explanations for all the major facts concerning heart attacks. These explanations relate all the observed phenomena back to certain measurable quantities with which we can deal confidently in understanding the problem for each individual.

In the course of presenting this information, some of the features concerning heart attacks that still require further clarification and understanding have also been pointed out so that the reader can know where some loopholes still do exist in our knowledge of the phenomenon of occurrence of heart attacks in our population. It would be folly to state that everything is known about heart attacks. This is definitely not the case. It is equally foolish to deny that a tremendous amount is known. Our task now is to consider such questions as "What can we do with the information that is already at our disposal to start preventing heart attacks *now*, or to treat them, if they have already occurred, in the hope of minimizing the chance of a second heart attack?" In essence this amounts to asking how we apply the fabulous knowledge that has been won by much hard effort in research and medical practice over the past hundred years. First, it can be stated that pitifully little is being done today in a practical way, contrasted with what could be done to cope with this major medical hazard of our time.

A real program for prevention of heart attacks in the United States on any reasonable scale involves two broad principles: (1) the effective application of what we know now to the problem of prevention of heart attacks in our population, and (2) the initiation of a really worthwhile and intensive effort to fill some of the gaps in our knowledge which would make any present program very much more effective.

The application of what we know now in the prevention of heart attacks

Primary to any consideration of prevention of heart attacks with what we now know is the determination of *who is in need of preventive efforts*. In reviewing the evidence concerning the prediction of heart attacks, it has been stressed that we have no direct way of knowing by usual types of medical examination whether or not a particular person's risk of having a heart attack at some future time is low, intermediate, or high. We know, for example, that a typical examination as practiced today by doctors including an electrocardiogram, with all the findings being pronounced normal, is in no way a safe assurance against a high risk of a heart attack. The underlying disease, hardening of the coronary arteries, goes on silently until it has produced a heart attack. None of the usual techniques of medical examination will tell us the crucial information concerning this person with the exception of one piece of evidence, his blood pressure. This one feature can be detected in a routine clinical examination. If the blood pressure is high, we do know that the risk of heart attack is increased.

But this is only one facet of the story, and in general not the most important one. The more important feature in determination of heart attack risk is the amount of certain fatty materials in the blood, known as lipoproteins, that amount being summarized in a measurement called the Atherogenic Index. All the evidence considered in this book—such as the greater incidence of heart attacks in young men than young women, the increasing frequency of heart attacks with increasing age, the occurrence of heart attacks in persons who habitually consume certain types of diets, the occurrence of heart attacks in the overweight, the occurrence of excessive heart attacks in cigarette smokers, the occurrence of excessive heart attacks in certain families, the relationship of occupation to heart attacks, the effects of life stresses—points to the crucial factors involved being the amount of blood lipoproteins and the level of the blood pressure.

People with increased risks of heart attacks as a result of one or another of a large variety of phenomena show such increased risks because of either an indirect effect in elevating the amount in the blood of certain of the lipoproteins, or an effect in the elevation of the blood pressure, or in some combination of both. It was shown clearly that the lipoproteins and the blood pressure provide separate information, that both factors are involved in heart disease risk, and that such risk can increase because of unfavorable values of either of these factors or of both. In some persons one factor is primarily involved, in other persons the second factor is involved, and in still others both are active.

In a determination of who is in need of prevention and, obviously, who can forget about the risk of future heart attacks, we need not use any of the indirect weaker evidence, such as the simple fact that the subject is a man rather than a woman.

Many men do not share the higher average risk of men in general. Therefore we should use instead the direct evidence which relates to heart attacks—the level of the blood lipoproteins and the level of the blood pressure. Since we cannot tell simply by looking at any man or woman in the population whether he or she is high in blood pressure or high in lipoprotein level, the only way to know the answer is to examine that particular man or woman to determine where he or she stands on these measurements. No one in the population is exempt from the possibility of having a high lipoprotein–Atherogenic Index value in the blood or of having a high blood pressure. This being the case, a really adequate program of prevention of heart attacks means that every adult above the age of twenty-five years deserves immediately to be checked to determine whether or not he falls into a category of a high risk of future coronary heart disease as a result of a high level of the lipoproteins in the blood or a high blood pressure, or both. Thereafter, on some periodic schedule such as every three to five years, every person should be rechecked with regard to his status concerning blood pressure and blood lipoproteins, to determine whether or not a favorable status originally determined is still being maintained. We know that, in the main, a favorable status will be maintained unless the person changes grossly his dietary habits, increases in weight, or develops some medical abnormality such as diabetes mellitus or an inadequate thyroid gland function.

Is any of this being done now? Not on anything like the scale that it needs to be done, if we are to apply the information we now have to identification of those in need of preventive measures for heart attacks. To be sure, it is being done to a minor extent. The technical means for making the necessary measurements of the lipoproteins of the blood and of the blood pressure are routine and available to every physician in the land. The facilities for such studies are being used by thousands of physicians for individuals in their medical practice.

Such facilities are being used by certain of our large industrial corporations in preventive medical checkups of their executives. Such facilities are being used to check the blood of many scientists and physicians who already understand the nature of the evidence and want, for themselves at least, to utilize what we know now in the effort to prevent heart disease. But these facilities are not being used on the scale that they should be— in checking every adult in the United States. Every adult is potentially a candidate for an excessive risk of coronary heart disease, and therefore every adult is in need of checking.

The reason for delay in doing precisely this is largely that medicine has in general been oriented to the problem of treatment, for adults at least. When a disease develops, the physician considers using the most efficacious means at his disposal for treating the person with that disease. With heart attacks, this approach is extremely late in the game. The real time for treatment is in the very early stages, when the narrowing of the coronary arteries begins and when it should properly be intercepted. In this way the risk of a heart attack five, ten, fifteen, or twenty years later can be avoided or at least minimized to a great extent. Industrial corporations recognize the tremendous value of preventive medicine for their leading executives.

Numerous such organizations have begun to incorporate the examination of the blood pressure and of the blood lipoproteins in an annual medical checkup of their top executives. Their view is that by identifying those carrying an excessive risk of heart disease, the major hazard to life in these individuals in any event, they can institute measures designed to alter the situation toward a more favorable outlook with a much smaller risk of future heart attacks. The economic and organizational value of an executive to a large industrial corporation and the value of an important military leader to a military organization are self-evident; and preventive measures are being actively pursued early for such groups.

But who is to measure the economic and human value of any individual in the population at large? Certainly to himself and to his family any individual is valuable enough to consider doing anything within reason to attempt to prevent his becoming an early victim of a heart attack. Yet, both from certain members of the public and the medical profession has come the complaint that to do this on a large scale, for every person in the population, would be very costly.

Let us analyze the general order of magnitude of the cost for the complete examinations that would be necessary to determine a person's status once every three to five years with respect to the risk of a future heart attack. On a broad basis, such costs would not conceivably be over twenty-five dollars per person for such an examination and in all probability would be less. If the examination were done every three to five years our cost would be between three and eight dollars per year per person in the population. It is very difficult to imagine how something approximating five dollars a year per person could be regarded either by members of the public or by members of the medical profession as a stumbling block to institution of a real program of preventive medicine for adults—a preventive medicine designed to counter the risk of the major killer of our time. It seems extremely difficult to measure the value of delaying a heart attack from age forty to age fifty or to age sixty in terms of two, five, ten, or fifteen dollars per year. Even if we considered this on a nation-wide basis for one hundred million adults, the entire cost of such examinations as a public service would run in the neighborhood of approximately $500,-000,000 per year—a small fraction of our annual defense budget. The author would be the first to state that we need strong defense, and if this requires forty billion dollars a year we should certainly spend forty billion dollars to achieve it. However, when we consider that heart attacks kill each year in our country numbers of our people comparable with the total number of deaths of Americans in World War II, it does not seem reasonable to state that $500,000,000 to institute an effective preventive medical program is a large sum of money in a land such as ours.

Undoubtedly, as the information concerning what we now know about heart attacks and what can be done to predict their risk spreads to the public and the medical profession, there will be an increasing pressure for an active widespread program to do something about this problem. Then, widespread examination of individuals, and ultimately every individual in the population, will become routine. The question is whether or not one would like to wait one, five, ten, or a hundred years with all the attendant unnecessary deaths occurring in the interim before an effective heart attack prevention program becomes a reality.

Let us assume that a broad program of prevention of heart attacks were instituted, incorporating the examination of the blood pressure and the examination of the amount of the blood lipoproteins in every adult over twenty-five years of age. How would we proceed with the information derived therefrom to try to prevent heart attacks? First of all, as a result of such examinations it would be possible to select out of the population a large number of people whose values are low, or moderately low. For such individuals the risk of future heart attacks is so low that it is hardly worth while concerning them any further about the problem. The major need for such persons is to reassure them that the risk of a heart attack is a minor problem, and that so long as their values remain in the low range they need do nothing about it, except possibly to have recheck determinations of their status made every three to five years. Such examinations of every adult in the population will also reveal some with high values either of the blood lipoproteins or blood pressure or both and who therefore carry an excessive risk of development of heart attacks in the future. This does not mean, nor has it ever been claimed by responsible sources to mean, that such individuals are definitely going to develop a heart attack in a one-, five-, or ten-year period. Indeed, unless the values are extremely high, the chances of avoiding a heart attack are better than those of having one. The real issue, however, is that such individuals may be two, five, ten, twenty, or more times the average in terms of their risk of having a heart attack. Prudence in their own hygiene would suggest that if any measures are available for reducing this excessive risk of heart disease they would want to take them.

This brings us to the question of what preventive measures now available can be expected to accomplish toward material reduction in the excessive risk of future heart attacks. Provision of a sensible answer to this question requires that we consider the picture as a whole, utilizing the best evidence on the subject at our disposal. First, we have the assured evidence that when either the lipoprotein or blood pressure values (or both) are high, the risk of coronary heart attacks is increased. It would seem eminently logical, then, that if these high values of the lipoproteins and blood pressure (which account for the high risk of heart disease) could be lowered and maintained lowered, the risk of future heart attack might be expected to drop back toward some lower value. This seems likely, from elementary reasoning. It is on this basis, indeed, that a vast majority of the physicians and research workers interested in heart disease are going ahead in the effort to develop a preventive medical approach for heart attacks.

However, the skeptical individual might say "Yes, I will grant that if the lipoprotein and blood pressure values are high, you have proved the case of a high risk of future heart attacks. How do I know in terms of actual proof that lowering these values will of itself lower the risk of heart attacks?" Their concern is over whether it *might be* that some third factor raises the blood lipoprotein and pressure values and also raises the heart attack risk. Lowering the lipoproteins and blood pressure might not accomplish the task of reducing the future heart attack risk if their hypothetical third factor is not also lowered (no evidence exists for such a third factor). There is a mass of direct evidence and auxiliary indirect evidence which suggests that these skeptics are worrying rather needlessly.

Let us return to the evidence concerning overweight individuals. Life insurance statistics have shown quite clearly that excessive overweight is associated with an increased heart attack risk. Most of this excessive heart disease risk due to overweight is associated with an elevation of the lipoproteins or the blood pressure, or both. We can now ask whether or not any information exists concerning proof of the benefit of correction of overweight. Such proof does exist. There were a certain number of life insurance policyholders who were overweight but who had the opportunity to qualify for a lower premium by reducing their weight. On analysis of the information concerning the fate of thousands of such policyholders who did lose weight to return their weight toward the ideal value, the life insurance statisticians found that such persons *lost* their excessive risk of development of heart disease. This is very powerful direct evidence which indicates that correcting the overweight, which would be expected to correct the lipoprotein elevation and the blood pressure elevation in part, at least, has produced the desired result of reducing the risk of heart attack mortality. If we remember further that the mechanism by which heart attack risk is raised in individuals who have high lipoprotein values and high blood pressure values is by the route of an acceleration of the rate at which their coronary arteries harden, can we anticipate that lowering of elevated lipoprotein and blood pressure values will slow this hardening process? Can we even possibly expect that some of the existing hardening of the coronary arteries may actually reverse itself with correction of the high lipoprotein or blood pressure values?

Here some special evidence is pertinent and extremely important. There exists a group of people who have extremely high values of the lipoproteins in the blood, the very same lipoproteins that exist in the blood of everyone else in variable amounts and which are associated with heart attack risk. In these special individuals (who, incidentally, have an extremely high death rate due to heart attacks) not only are the lipoprotein values high enough to cause them to form the hardening deposits in their coronary arteries, but they are also high enough to form very similar deposits in tissues such as the skin. These deposits in the skin have been named xanthomas, yellow lumps. Microscopically, these lumps are extremely similar to the hardened deposits in the coronary arteries and in all probability represent an analogous disease in the skin, occurring only with very high levels of the lipoproteins in the blood. It appears that in general the skin is less likely as an organ to receive such deposits, and in the population at large, where the lipoprotein levels are not nearly so high, even though the arteries develop these hardening deposits the skin does not. However, in these selected individuals with extremely high levels of the lipoproteins, not only do the arterial deposits develop but also the skin deposits develop. Such persons provide an excellent way to study the value of lowering the blood lipoproteins, for their deposits in the skin are directly visible, measurable, and can be felt. What will be the fate of such skin deposits, if the lipoproteins of the blood are successfully lowered in amount? This has now been tested in over a dozen patients with large areas of these skin deposits of varying duration. By making use of the information (see Chapter 10) that animal (or saturated) fat restriction will lower elevated S_f 0–20 lipoprotein levels and that carbohydrate restriction will lower S_f 20–400 lipoprotein levels, it was readily possible to design diets for these patients so that their elevation in lipoprotein levels was materially corrected—toward much lower levels. These patients have been under observation for many months, some of them for several years. In every case of this type that has been studied the following important facts have been found.

First, whereas the person was going on to develop new lumps in the skin *before* the lipoproteins were lowered, and to show an increase in the size of older lumps in the skin, *no such new lumps* and *no increase in the size of existing lumps were ob*-served when the lipoprotein levels were brought down and kept down by dietary means.

Second, in most of these individuals not only did new lumps fail to appear but *the older lumps gradually lost some of the fatty material from them, gradually shrank in size, and in many instances even disappeared entirely!* Thus a deposit extremely similar to the deposit in the coronary arteries, visible to the naked eye and directly measurable, is observed to undergo precisely the changes one would hope to observe under the influence of a marked lowering of the blood lipoprotein levels. Logic would have led us to expect that since the high level of lipoproteins is associated with deposition, lowering the levels of lipoproteins should at least arrest new deposition. This was observed. Indeed, it was much more than had been hoped for to observe that the deposits which had already been formed either shrank in size markedly or disappeared entirely.

The process of deposition and hardening that goes on in the coronary artery is extremely similar to that in the skin. There is excellent reason to believe that perhaps at a lesser, perhaps at a greater, rate a similar arrest in new deposition and a decrease in size of old deposits would both occur, with a lowering in the blood lipoproteins or a lowering of the blood pressure, or both. A valuable lesson has also been learned from the deposits that occur in these skin xanthomas, or yellow lumps. It was noted in many of the individuals with these deposits in the skin that some of them had been there for three, five, or seven years but others had been of recent origin, a few months or a year. The deposits of recent origin, less than a year or so in duration, were the quickest to decrease in size and most often disappeared entirely with treatment. In contrast, the deposits that had been present for a period of many years decreased in size but did not disappear entirely. They left a residue of scarred, fibrous tissue that apparently had developed as a result of the long existence of the fatty deposits. We know from the development of the similar disease in the arteries that such scarred, fibrous areas occur there, too. What this teaches us is that even if we institute a program to stop new deposition and to reverse old deposition in coronary arteries, the longer deposition has been there the greater the chance there will be for more of the fibrous elements of the hardening and the lower will be the chance of removing it. This points up the real need to intercept this process early in its development. If we wait until there has been a large conversion to the fibrous, hardened material in the artery, there is a good possibility that we will not be able to do much about this part of the disease.

Evidence has been brought to bear on this problem from still other sources. Although the human differs vastly from experimental animals such as the dog—in which hardening of the arteries has been produced by certain special diets—and although we can not by any means extrapolate from the dog to the human, we certainly cannot close our eyes to the evidence derived from animal experiment. In the dog, hardening of the arteries is produced by a special diet which raises the blood lipoproteins. If the diet is then restored to a usual one for the dog, the lipoprotein levels fall back to normal. After a period of months on the normal diet it is found that the hardening of the arteries which would have been there, had the animals been sacrificed at the time the special diet was stopped, has actually regressed and even disappeared in many areas. This agrees with the human evidence for the skin lumps: not only does new hardening cease when the lipoprotein levels are lowered but also old hardening is in large measure reversed. This is further powerful evidence in favor of the logic of lowering the lipoprotein levels in order to stop new disease and reverse old disease. While such evidence is derived in the dog, it is almost certainly applicable, at least in a modified sense, to the human case.

Also, in recent years a great deal of research by pharmaceutical companies and by university pharmacology and clinical medical departments has been done on drugs of various sorts that are capable of reducing elevated blood pressures. While all the observations are not so carefully controlled as one would like, it appears inescapable, from the experience of a vast number of clinics working with these drugs, that individuals whose high blood pressures have been lowered are definitely experiencing a lowering of the incidence of heart disease as compared with the period before such drugs were available. This again is rather direct evidence that the mortality risk is lowered by reducing one of the major factors associated with heart disease, if that factor is elevated. All the evidence, direct and indirect, and all the logic point to the value of reducing the lipoproteins, when elevated, and the blood pressure, when elevated, in the effort to minimize the risk of future heart attacks. To be sure, further evidence on large human groups would be desirable supplementary information, but it is by no means necessary to await this before going ahead with a highly reasonable program for prevention of heart attacks now.

Such supplemental information could come in one of two ways. First, if the entire population of the United States were brought into a preventive medical program, their lipoprotein and blood pressure values determined, and every effort made to lower elevated values by dietary, pharmaceutical, and other means at our disposal now, one need simply observe the heart attack rate, which has been on the increase over the last few decades in this country. If that heart attack rate trend reversed itself and started down, this in itself would be evidence that the measures had been effective. This, of course, is a very large-scale endeavor and would probably take a fair amount of time to accomplish.

A shorter way to this goal would be to take a group of individuals, as many as ten or twenty thousand persons, who have high values of the heart attack risk because of high lipoprotein values and high blood pressures and to divide such a group into two equal subgroups. One group could be observed without any treatment. In the other group all reasonable measures for reducing elevated lipoprotein levels or elevated blood pressures or both could be applied. With careful observation of these two groups, within a matter of one to two years one could expect that if the measures are effective, as all the evidence indicates they would be, there should be a pronounced difference in the heart attack rate between the two groups. This is, too, a large-scale experiment, requiring the cooperation of many thousands of individuals and some hard work by those who organize and conduct the experiment. It might also cost a fair sum of money, but an amount of money which would be trivial in comparison with the goal and results that are being sought. The American public is keenly aware of the real problem of heart disease and undoubtedly would lend a full measure of cooperation to an experiment such as this—which, if well conducted, would lead to such crucial answers. It is pathetic that inertia has so far prevented such a study from being undertaken and carried through to completion.

In part, the study has not been done because it would require a large amount of public cooperation and this would involve a large amount of explanation to the public of what one is trying to accomplish. The fear has existed in the minds of some that the public could not possibly understand the problem and would not be helpful. The author does not subscribe to this at all. The public is highly intelligent, highly concerned about this problem, and certainly would go to very great lengths in the effort to help once and for all to determine directly and quickly what a particular measure would do in the way of reducing the heart attack risk. Indeed, this seems to be one of the best ways of getting the information in a direct way, which would be highly worth while.

With respect to the measures available for accomplishing the reduction of elevated lipoprotein and Atherogenic Index values, and hence in the heart attack risk, many are now at our disposal and can be used by those who are endeavoring to reduce their risk. The application of these measures can be most intelligently achieved through the careful cooperation of a physician and the individual he cares for medically in the effort to prevent heart attacks. Those individuals who have been studied and found to have high levels of the lipoproteins, primarily of the S_f 0–20 class, require one type of management. This is the group of lipoproteins that is elevated, on the average, by diets containing high amounts of animal fats, or saturated vegetable fats. In such individuals it has been proved by the work of many laboratories that these lipoprotein levels can be lowered if the individual reduces the dietary intake of such animal and saturated vegetable fats. Since the liquid, or unsaturated, vegetable oils do not have this effect of raising S_f 0–20 lipoprotein levels, the substitution of them for the animal and saturated vegetable fats removed helps provide a palatable, satisfying, and enjoyable diet. Such a dietary modification will, in general, lower elevated S_f 0–20 lipoprotein levels. On the other hand, there exist many individuals whose heart attack risk does not come from the S_f 0–20 lipoproteins primarily but rather from the elevation in level of S_f 20–400 lipoproteins.

In such individuals it has been proved that high levels of S_f 20–400 lipoproteins can be produced, on the average, by a high intake of carbohydrates and that the levels can be lowered if the person reduces the dietary carbohydrate intake. These are long-term effects on humans, tested carefully on one type of diet against another, in this country under the usual circumstances of living. If they are not overweight, such individuals can replace the caloric value of the carbohydrates they have removed by supplementation of their diet with one of the liquid vegetable oils which will do nothing to raise their lipoprotein values. The supplementation of the diet with vegetable oil, whether to replace animal fat or carbohydrates or both, provides a highly nutritious, satisfying diet, without any real deprivation on the part of the person. The principles of such dieting, including menus, recipes, and precise amounts of the various foodstuffs that should be eaten, have been described in great detail in the book entitled *The Dietary Prevention and Treatment of Heart Disease* by the author and his colleagues.* It would require a volume to repeat all that information here.

The major point is that the principles of dieting in an effort to lower these lipoprotein classes and thereby to lower the risk of heart disease have been abundantly described, together with very practical daily cooking menus and recipes that have been kitchen-tested on persons who have been on these diets for periods of months and years. There is no evidence whatever that these diets restricted in animal fat intake or carbohydrate intake can do any harm or in any way unfavorably influence the health of individuals. Such diets can be made completely adequate, and more than adequate, in all the known essential nutrients recommended by the National Research Council. A large number of physicians are advising patients to reduce their animal and saturated vegetable fat intake and their carbohydrate intake with the replacement of some of the calories lost with unsaturated, liquid vegetable oil even though these patients have not been evaluated for their lipoprotein status. This is done on the general principle that if the patients are taking in much more animal fat or carbohydrates than they need, it would be the better part of wisdom to modify their diet toward one which might be recommended to prevent lipoprotein elevation. The only thing one can say about this is that while it is in the right direction, it is somewhat hit-or-miss in that there are many individuals who will diet needlessly. If the lipoproteins are already low, there is no need to try to reduce them further. Also, with this "blind" procedure, an individual will not know whether he should be concentrating more on the side of reduction of animal fat intake than on the side of reduction of carbohydrate intake. In addition to dietary measures, certain pharmaceutical substances can now be prescribed by physicians

* *The Dietary Prevention and Treatment of Heart Disease* by John W. Gofman, Alex V. Nichols, and Virginia Dobbin (New York: G. P. Putnam's Sons, Inc., 1958).

to aid many patients in their efforts to reduce elevated S_f 0–20 or S_f 20–400 lipoprotein levels.

Secondly, under medical supervision, elevated blood pressure should be reduced wherever it is possible to do so. The pharmaceutical agents required for the reduction of blood pressure should not be used by an individual without medical supervision. However, the principle of reduction of elevated blood pressure even if it is causing no obvious difficulty at the moment should definitely be followed, for we know that the elevated blood pressure is producing an excessive risk of future heart attacks by increasing the rate at which the coronary arteries are hardening. So much for the immediate program of what we can do now with our present knowledge in the effort to prevent heart attacks.

The initiation of efforts to fill the gaps in our existing knowledge

While a great deal can and should be done immediately to start a widespread preventive medicine program to reduce heart attack rates, there exists an even more important horizon. It has been pointed out in this book that many of the findings are quoted to be true "on the average." Thus, on the average, the lipoproteins of the S_f 0–20 class will rise in level when the dietary intake of animal, or saturated, fat is high. Or, on the average, the S_f 20–400 lipoprotein levels will be high when the dietary intake of carbohydrates is high. On the average, overweight is associated with an elevation of lipoproteins and Atherogenic Index values. This in essence is another way of stating that not all individuals respond alike to the dietary factors or to alterations in body weight. Individuals are quite variable with respect to the amount of the various lipoproteins they will have in their blood under a particular set of conditions. Thus, while it is certainly true that one individual may experience a large rise in his S_f 20–400 lipoprotein level with the daily consumption of 400 grams of carbohydrates, it is also true that another individual of the same sex and age might experience only a very slight rise while eating exactly the same amount of carbohydrates during a test period.

We know that for people in the population at large, at a given age and for one sex, individuals range from the very low blood levels of the lipoproteins up to very high levels. At low lipoprotein values, we can find some individuals who are consuming much more of the foods that we know can raise lipoprotein levels than some of the people who have very high values of the same lipoprotein classes. Even though, for those who have high lipoprotein levels when they consume a particular type of diet, very beneficial results can be achieved by alteration of that diet, we also know that other individuals can consume even greater excesses of this diet without showing high lipoprotein levels. This is the crucial feature of the entire problem and the feature which deserves investigation very urgently. Why is it that certain people in the population have low levels of the lipoproteins with our usual diets while others have intermediate levels, and still others have high levels? This is of course related to the question of why it is that men have, in general, higher lipoprotein levels than women at least in early adult life. It is one matter to describe this difference in lipoprotein levels between men and women; it is quite another matter to understand the basis for it. Why any individual is characterized by a certain lipoprotein value on a particular type of diet usual in our country is one of the most important questions that future research in heart disease could answer.

There is every need for a concerted effort to ferret out the basis in bodily biochemistry for the ability of certain individuals to handle nearly any type of food without elevation of their lipoprotein levels. Today, and for highly practical purposes, we must consider the use of diets altered in animal fat intake or diets altered in carbohydrate intake in order to reduce heart attack risk in persons with high lipoprotein levels. But the real future of the effort to prevent heart disease lies in understanding how it is that we might possibly convert the person who does not handle the foods well to be more like the person who does. This problem seems very definitely to be one of fundamental body chemistry. There is no reason to regard this as a problem that is outside the pale of ordinary biochemistry, or as one that cannot be solved. We can grant that a great deal of work and research may be required for its solution. No problem concerning the field of heart disease and heart attacks could be said to be more important than that of determining why a particular person has a low, intermediate, or high level of the major lipoprotein classes and the Atherogenic Index. Some efforts are going into this problem in the form of studies of the effect of various drugs, and in the form of studies of the relationship of some of the lipoproteins to each other and to other biochemical features of the person, but the national effort on this problem at the present time is not a concerted one.

A really concerted effort is urgently needed. If a team of 100 or more of the top medical scientists in the country devoting their effort completely to this one problem were to spend five or ten years on it, undoubtedly some major answers would come forth. The cost of this type of effort would be trivial in terms of the stakes with which we are dealing. Since the lipoprotein levels are a major factor in determining the risk of heart attacks, any additional understanding we can achieve, at a fundamental biochemical level, of why they are high when they are high is of tremendous value. Such knowledge would undoubtedly greatly increase our ability to lower elevated lipoprotein levels more efficiently than we now can. This is certainly a fabulous opportunity to work toward the goal of eliminating heart attacks from our population. Toward this goal, no amount of effort could conceivably be too much.